High Blood Pressure

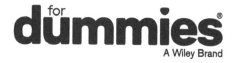

for
dummies®
A Wiley Brand

High Blood Pressure

3rd Edition

by Richard W. Snyder, DO,
with Alan L. Rubin, MD

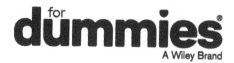

High Blood Pressure For Dummies®, 3rd Edition

Published by: **John Wiley & Sons, Inc.,** 111 River Street, Hoboken, NJ 07030-5774, www.wiley.com

Copyright © 2024 by John Wiley & Sons, Inc., Hoboken, New Jersey

Media and software compilation copyright © 2024 by John Wiley & Sons, Inc. All rights reserved.

Published simultaneously in Canada

For general information on our other products and services, please contact our Customer Care Department within the U.S. at 877-762-2974, outside the U.S. at 317-572-3993, or fax 317-572-4002. For technical support, please visit https://hub.wiley.com/community/support/dummies.

Wiley publishes in a variety of print and electronic formats and by print-on-demand. Some material included with standard print versions of this book may not be included in e-books or in print-on-demand. If this book refers to media such as a CD or DVD that is not included in the version you purchased, you may download this material at http://booksupport.wiley.com. For more information about Wiley products, visit www.wiley.com.

Library of Congress Control Number: 2023951014

ISBN 978-1-394-22494-4 (pbk); ISBN 978-1-394-22496-8 (ebk); ISBN 978-1-394-22495-1 (ebk)

SKY10061971_120623

Contents at a Glance

Introduction 1

Part 1: Understanding High Blood Pressure 5
CHAPTER 1: Introducing High Blood Pressure 7
CHAPTER 2: Detecting High Blood Pressure 13
CHAPTER 3: Determining Whether You're at Risk 23
CHAPTER 4: Reviewing the Causes of Resistant High Blood Pressure 29

Part 2: Considering the Medical Consequences of High Blood Pressure 49
CHAPTER 5: Protecting Your Heart from Heart Disease 51
CHAPTER 6: Caring for Your Kidneys 69
CHAPTER 7: Keeping Your Brain Intact 87
CHAPTER 8: Eyeing Your Blood Pressure 101

Part 3: Preventing and Treating High Blood Pressure 105
CHAPTER 9: Choosing Foods That Lower High Blood Pressure 107
CHAPTER 10: Keeping Salt and Sugar Out of Your Diet 121
CHAPTER 11: Avoiding Tobacco, Alcohol, and Caffeine 129
CHAPTER 12: Lowering Blood Pressure with Exercise 141
CHAPTER 13: Taking Medications to Lower Your Blood Pressure 153
CHAPTER 14: Considering Important Clinical Studies of High Blood Pressure 185

Part 4: Taking Care of Special Populations 191
CHAPTER 15: Handling High Blood Pressure in Older Adults 193
CHAPTER 16: Handling High Blood Pressure in Children 203
CHAPTER 17: Treating High Blood Pressure in Women 211

Part 5: The Part of Tens 221
CHAPTER 18: Ten Simple Ways to Prevent or Reduce High Blood Pressure 223
CHAPTER 19: Ten (or So) Myths about High Blood Pressure 231

Appendix: Resources 239

Index 243

Table of Contents

INTRODUCTION 1

About This Book. 1

Foolish Assumptions. 2

Icons Used in This Book 2

Beyond the Book. 3

Where to Go from Here 3

PART 1: UNDERSTANDING HIGH BLOOD PRESSURE 5

CHAPTER 1: **Introducing High Blood Pressure** 7

Understanding Your Cardiovascular System. 8

Measuring Your Blood Pressure and Understanding the
Measurement. 8

Looking at the Risk Factors for High Blood Pressure. 9

Focusing on the Consequences of High Blood Pressure. 10

Lowering High Blood Pressure with Different Treatments 10

Evaluating High Blood Pressure in Children, Women,
and Older People. 11

CHAPTER 2: **Detecting High Blood Pressure**. 13

Looking at the Gauge Used to Measure Blood Pressure. 14

Taking Your Blood Pressure Correctly 15

Understanding the Numbers. 18

Lowering Blood Pressure Too Much. 19

Getting the Right Assessment 20

Reviewing your history 21

Having a physical exam 21

Looking at lab tests 22

CHAPTER 3: **Determining Whether You're at Risk**. 23

Reviewing Important Aspects of High Blood Pressure 24

Understanding the effect of genetics. 25

Estimating the effects of ethnicity. 25

Seeing how medication can affect blood pressure 26

Changing Your Lifestyle to Prevent High Blood Pressure 26

CHAPTER 4: **Reviewing the Causes of Resistant High
Blood Pressure** 29

Identifying the Signs and Symptoms of Resistant
High Blood Pressure 30

Considering Chronic Kidney Disease and High Blood Pressure. . . . 31

Navigating Narrowed Renal Arteries 32
    Diagnosing renal artery stenosis. 33
    Treating blocked renal arteries 34
Homing in on Hormones That Cause Hypertension 36
    Finding an epinephrine-producing tumor 37
    Detecting a tumor that produces aldosterone 39
    Recognizing Cushing's syndrome 43
Evaluating Other Causes of Resistant High Blood Pressure 46
    Coarctation of the aorta. 46
    Too much or too little thyroid hormone .47
    Sleep apnea 47

PART 2: CONSIDERING THE MEDICAL CONSEQUENCES OF HIGH BLOOD PRESSURE

PART 2: CONSIDERING THE MEDICAL CONSEQUENCES
OF HIGH BLOOD PRESSURE 49

CHAPTER 5: **Protecting Your Heart from Heart Disease** 51
    Introducing the Mighty Heart: Pumping and Relaxing. 52
    Blocking Blood Flow to the Heart Muscle .53
    Analyzing Coronary Artery Disease. 56
        Understanding angina and heart attack 57
        Getting a diagnosis 58
        Considering treatment options. 60
    Developing Congestive Heart Failure 62
        Noticing important signs and symptoms. 62
        Understanding what your doctor will look for 63
        Determining the underlying cause of heart failure 63
        Treating congestive heart failure 65
    Recognizing and Treating Important Risk Factors 65
        Reducing high cholesterol 66
        Quitting smoking. 66
        Controlling diabetes 66
        Stepping up physical activity 67

CHAPTER 6: **Caring for Your Kidneys** 69
    Examining the Role of Your Kidneys. 70
        Filtering. 71
        Making hormones 72
    Understanding Chronic Kidney Disease and Common Causes 73
        Defining chronic kidney disease 74
        Diagnosing chronic kidney disease. 74
        Staging and treating chronic kidney disease. 75
    Coping with End-Stage Renal Disease 76
        Dialysis 77
        Kidney transplant 82

CHAPTER 7: **Keeping Your Brain Intact**. 87
    Understanding the Causes of Strokes 88
        Atherosclerosis 88
        Cerebral embolus 89
        Brain hemorrhage. 90
    Preventing Stroke 91
        Understanding the risk factors you can't change. 92
        Modifying the risk factors you can 92
        Reducing stroke risk with medications. 93
    Thinking F.A.S.T. When Suspecting a Stroke 94
    Utilizing Brain Imaging 95
    Understanding Treatment Options for Stroke 97
    Recovering from a Stroke. 98
        Regaining function. 98
        Working with rehabilitation specialists 98

CHAPTER 8: **Eyeing Your Blood Pressure**. 101
    Eyeballing the Anatomy of the Eye 102
    Getting Hyper about Hypertensive Retinopathy. 103

PART 3: PREVENTING AND TREATING HIGH
BLOOD PRESSURE 105

CHAPTER 9: **Choosing Foods That Lower High
    Blood Pressure** 107
    DASHing Down Your Blood Pressure 108
        Leading up to DASH 108
        Proving the value of DASH. 109
        Getting with the program. 110
        Reducing your salt consumption with DASH. 113
    Maximizing the Mediterranean Diet to Lower Your
    Blood Pressure. 114
    Seeing the Value of a Plant-Based Diet Plan 115
    Losing Weight with Nutrition. 115
        Calculating your ideal weight. 116
        Determining your daily caloric needs. 116
        Adjusting your DASH nutrition plan .118
    Consulting with a Nutritionist 120

CHAPTER 10: **Keeping Salt and Sugar Out of Your Diet** 121
    Making the Connection between Salt and High Blood Pressure 121
        Proving the connection between sodium and high
        blood pressure. 122

Looking at salt sensitivity 123
Lowering your salt intake 124
Connecting Sugar and High Blood Pressure: The Role of Insulin 127

CHAPTER 11: **Avoiding Tobacco, Alcohol, and Caffeine** 129
Playing with Fire: Tobacco and High Blood Pressure 130
Examining the extent of the problem 130
Understanding the consequences of tobacco use 131
Reducing your exposure to secondhand smoke 131
Avoiding all forms of tobacco 132
Quitting tobacco successfully 133
Tapping into resources 136
Linking Alcohol to High Blood Pressure 136
Cutting Back on Caffeine 137
Knowing how much is too much 138
Considering caffeine's health consequences 139
Recognizing the gains in giving up caffeine 139
Avoiding the beans, chocolate, energy drinks, and soda 139

CHAPTER 12: **Lowering Blood Pressure with Exercise** 141
Recognizing the Benefits of Exercise 142
Preparing to Begin an Exercise Program 142
Getting a checkup 143
Personalizing your exercise program 144
Using the right equipment 147
Exercising to Lose Weight 148
Exercising to Gain Strength 149
Lowering Your Blood Pressure with Complementary Therapies 149
Yoga 150
Meditation 150
Biofeedback 151

CHAPTER 13: **Taking Medications to Lower Your Blood
Pressure** 153
Examining Classes of Blood Pressure Medications 154
Diuretics: Medications that reduce fluid buildup 155
Other first-line medications 162
Medications that act on the nervous system 170
Vasodilators: Medications that open the blood vessels 175
Choosing the Right Medication 177
Reviewing basic principles of medication dosing 177
Personalizing the medication choice 178
Selecting another medication when necessary 178
Adhering to the medication prescription 179

Recognizing Common Medication Side Effects 179
Identifying Brand Names 182

CHAPTER 14: **Considering Important Clinical Studies of High Blood Pressure** 185
SPRINT: Systolic Blood Pressure Intervention Trial 186
STEP: Strategy of Blood Pressure Intervention in the Elderly
Hypertensive Patients. 187
ACCORD: Action to Control Cardiovascular Risk in Diabetes 188
ADVANCE: Action in Diabetes and Vascular Disease 189

PART 4: TAKING CARE OF SPECIAL POPULATIONS 191

CHAPTER 15: **Handling High Blood Pressure in Older Adults** 193
Evaluating Cognitive Ability 194
Assessing Blood Pressure in an Older Person 195
Recognizing baseline high blood pressure 195
Considering resistant high blood pressure 196
Examining the medications that raise blood pressure 197
Improving Nutrition to Lower Blood Pressure 197
Assessing your nutritional status 198
Following the DASH nutrition plan 199
Reducing salt intake 199
Modifying Your Lifestyle to Lower Blood Pressure. 200
Taking Prescription Medications to Lower Blood Pressure. 200
Avoiding Dangerous Falls in Blood Pressure. 201

CHAPTER 16: **Handling High Blood Pressure in Children** 203
Measuring Blood Pressure and Interpreting the Results 204
Taking a blood pressure reading on tiny arms 204
Interpreting the results of the measurement 205
Considering the Causes of Elevated Blood Pressure 206
Surveying hereditary influences 206
Factoring in weight 207
Evaluating other possible causes 207
Initiating Treatment with Lifestyle Changes 208
Using Medications. 210

CHAPTER 17: **Treating High Blood Pressure in Women** 211
Connecting High Blood Pressure and Salt Sensitivity in Women 212
Understanding High Blood Pressure and Pregnancy. 212
Knowing what causes high blood pressure during pregnancy. . .213
Dealing with high blood pressure after delivery. 217

Using Hormone Treatments If You Have High Blood Pressure 218
Oral contraceptives. 218
Hormone replacement therapy. 219

PART 5: THE PART OF TENS. 221

CHAPTER 18: **Ten Simple Ways to Prevent or Reduce
High Blood Pressure**. 223
Know Your Blood Pressure 223
Know Whether You Have Resistant High Blood Pressure. 224
Adopt the DASH Diet. 225
Cut Out the Caffeine 225
Reduce the Amount of Salt in Your Diet. .226
Give Up Tobacco and Alcohol 227
Start an Exercise Program 227
Practice Mind-Body Techniques 228
Take Your Medication. 229
Avoid Medications That Raise Blood Pressure 229

CHAPTER 19: **Ten (or So) Myths about High Blood Pressure** 231
High Blood Pressure Is Inevitable as You Get Older 231
The Treatment Is Worse Than the Disease 232
You Must Restrict Your Life Because You Have High
Blood Pressure. 233
You Only Need Treatment If You Have High Systolic
Blood Pressure. 234
If You Have High Blood Pressure, You'll Have to Take
Medication Forever 234
You Can Stop Treatment after a Heart Attack or Stroke 235
You Should Avoid Exercise If You Have High Blood Pressure. 235
If You're Feeling Good, You Can Stop Taking Your
Blood Pressure Meds 236
High Blood Pressure Can't Be Controlled .236
People with High Blood Pressure Are Just Nervous or Anxious 237
Older People Don't Need to Be Treated. 237
High Blood Pressure Is Less Dangerous in Women. 238

APPENDIX: RESOURCES 239

INDEX. 243

Introduction

High blood pressure, technically known as *hypertension*, affects approximately 120 million people in the United States, according to the Centers for Disease Control and Prevention (CDC). That's roughly half of all adults in the United States!

High blood pressure doesn't usually have any symptoms, which means you can have high blood pressure for many years without even knowing it . . . until it's too late. That's why high blood pressure is known as the "silent killer." In addition to shortening your life span, high blood pressure affects several organs in the body, including the heart, brain, kidneys, and eyes.

In this book, you can find everything you need to know about high blood pressure — its causes, its consequences, and its treatment. You'll begin to realize that high blood pressure is easy to identify and just as easy to treat. An important aspect of treatment is prevention — changing your lifestyle habits to prevent high blood pressure from occurring in the first place.

About This Book

Since the last edition of this book, doctors have learned a lot about high blood pressure and its treatment. The categories of high blood pressure have changed and our recommendations for treatment have changed as well. We have more information about genetics and environmental influences, and significant clinical trials have dramatically affected our treatment of high blood pressure. We cover all this new information in this book. We also continue to emphasize prevention — with the information in this book, you can make simple changes to prevent or reverse high blood pressure so you never have to face the serious negative consequences that high blood pressure can have when it's left untreated.

Within this book, you may note that some web addresses break across two lines of text. If you're reading this book in print and want to visit one of these web pages, simply key in the web address exactly as it's noted in the text, pretending as though the line break doesn't exist. If you're reading this as an e-book, you've got it easy — just click the web address to be taken directly to the web page.

Foolish Assumptions

This book makes no assumptions about what you know regarding high blood pressure. If you're reading this book, you probably fall into one of the following categories:

>> You've been diagnosed with high blood pressure, but you haven't started treatment.

>> You're being treated for high blood pressure, but you aren't happy with the results.

>> You have a close friend or family member with high blood pressure.

Icons Used in This Book

Books in the *For Dummies* series feature icons that direct you toward information of particular interest or importance. Here's an explanation of this book's icons:

This icon means the information is essential. Be sure you understand it.

This icon points out important information that can save you time and improve your health.

The Technical Stuff icon marks information of a highly technical nature that you can normally skip over.

Take this icon seriously. It warns against potential problems (for example, being aware of medication side effects).

Beyond the Book

In addition to the abundance of information and guidance related to high blood pressure that we provide in this book, you get access to even more help and information online at Dummies.com. Check out this book's online Cheat Sheet. Just go to www.dummies.com and type **High Blood Pressure For Dummies Cheat Sheet** in the Search box.

Where to Go from Here

Where you go from here depends on what you want to read about. Do you want to understand how high blood pressure develops? Head to Part 1. If you or someone you know has a complication due to high blood pressure, skip to Part 2. For help in treating high blood pressure (or preventing it entirely), turn to Part 3. If you're pregnant or you have a child or parent with high blood pressure, Part 4 is your next stop. For a bird's-eye view of treatment and high blood pressure myths that need to be dispelled, check out Part 5.

We hope you find this book informative and enjoyable. Happy reading!

1

Understanding High Blood Pressure

IN THIS PART . . .

Understand those two numbers your doctor gives you after measuring your blood pressure.

Review the correct technique for measuring your blood pressure at home or at your doctor's office.

Find out who is at increased risk for developing high blood pressure.

Identify the causes of resistant high blood pressure.

Chapter **1**

Introducing High Blood Pressure

I f you have high blood pressure, you're not alone. According to the U.S. Centers for Disease Control and Prevention (CDC), approximately 120 million Americans have high blood pressure, which is defined as either taking prescribed medication for blood pressure or having blood pressure greater than 130/80. High blood pressure is a significant risk factor for heart attack, stroke, and vascular disease (see Part 2 of this book for more on these conditions).

You can do a lot to prevent high blood pressure or to lower it if you already have it. But before you act, you need to know what high blood pressure is and how you measure it. You also need to understand its causes and how it can be treated. This book is your blood pressure companion, providing you with a solid understanding of your blood pressure: how it affects your body organ by organ, who is at risk, how you can prevent it, and how you can treat it after it's properly diagnosed.

Understanding Your Cardiovascular System

To understand how high blood pressure affects your overall health, you need to understand the cardiovascular system — your heart, arteries, veins, capillaries, and the blood that fills them. The cardiovascular system carries

» **Nutrients** (carbohydrates, protein, fat, vitamins, and minerals) from the gastrointestinal tract to every organ in the body

» **Oxygen** from the lungs and in the blood to distant organs

» **Waste products,** a normal product of your body's metabolism (for example, carbon dioxide to the lungs and the other waste products to the liver and kidneys)

REMEMBER

Pressure must exist to push the blood through the cardiovascular system. (Otherwise your blood would pool in your legs due to gravity when you stood up!) Just as your household water supply reaches a faucet because of pressure pushing it through the pipes, blood reaches your brain because pressure is allowing it to defy gravity and rise from the heart.

The heart muscle (the source of this pressure) squeezes out the blood forcefully so the blood not only defies gravity but also travels through the smallest passageways (the *capillaries*, which are very small blood vessels in the body).

When essential body organs like the kidneys don't receive enough pressure to function properly, they signal the heart to pump harder. The sustained effect of high blood pressure over time is what's damaging to the brain, the blood vessels, and even the kidneys themselves. And that's when the consequences of high blood pressure occur (see Part 2).

Measuring Your Blood Pressure and Understanding the Measurement

When the medical staff in your health-care provider's office measure your blood pressure, they're using an automated blood pressure machine with a cuff wrapped around your arm. They press a button and wait while the automated blood pressure cuff squeezes your arm and measures your blood pressure. After a short amount of time, two numbers are displayed on the screen of the blood pressure machine, and these numbers are then recorded in your patient chart as part of your electronic medical record.

What do those numbers mean? When your health-care provider reads the numbers — say "135 over 85" — the first number is the *systolic blood pressure*, and the second number is the *diastolic blood pressure*. In Chapter 2, I explain what these blood pressure measurements mean and why the results have such a serious effect on your life.

TIP

One of the most effective steps you can take in understanding your health is to measure your own blood pressure with a home monitoring device. I cover this subject in Chapter 2 as well.

Looking at the Risk Factors for High Blood Pressure

Significant research has been done into the causes of high blood pressure, including genetic aspects and environmental influences (see Chapter 3). Numerous unalterable factors affect blood pressure, including age, gender, ethnic background, and family history.

The risk factors you *can* change (including diet, exercise, and stress) can also increase your risk of developing high blood pressure. Your health-care provider will likely ask you the following questions as part of an annual health assessment:

>> Are you less active than you could be in your day-to-day routine?

>> Are you overweight?

>> Do you consume foods high in salt and/or sugar?

>> Do you lead a stressful lifestyle?

>> Do you smoke and/or consume alcohol?

REMEMBER

If you answer "yes" to any one of these questions, you're at risk of developing high blood pressure. The more questions you answer "yes" to, the greater your odds of developing high blood pressure. On the other hand, if you're able to decrease the stress in your life and improve on some of these modifiable risk factors, you'll decrease your chances of developing high blood pressure.

The majority of high blood pressure in adults has been categorized as *essential high blood pressure* (blood pressure that occurs without an identifiable cause). We're learning more and more about the genetic influences of high blood pressure (see Chapter 3), as well *resistant* (very difficult to treat) causes of high blood pressure, including a condition called *hyperaldosteronism*, which may impact more cases of high blood pressure than previously thought. This and other causes of resistant high blood pressure are discussed in Chapter 4.

Focusing on the Consequences of High Blood Pressure

Left untreated, over time your high blood pressure can cause damage to your heart, kidneys, brain, and eyes:

>> Heart attacks or heart failure may be the major consequence for your heart (see Chapter 5).

>> Kidney disease can affect the filtering function of your kidneys, as well as itself be a cause of difficult-to-control high blood pressure (see Chapter 6).

>> An acute stroke may destroy important brain tissue and the movements it controls in the body (see Chapter 7).

>> The eyes are not the just the windows to the soul — they're also affected by uncontrolled blood pressure. Looking at the vessels in the eyes can be a clue that you have uncontrolled high blood pressure (see Chapter 8).

High blood pressure is the silent killer and these conditions are very much preventable. This book provides you with the tools you need to keep your blood pressure in check.

Lowering High Blood Pressure with Different Treatments

Treating high blood pressure (or preventing it entirely) involves all the tools I discuss in Part 3. Get started with the following guidelines, and check out Part 3 for an outline of a successful plan:

1. **Switch from a nutrition plan that promotes high blood pressure to a diet that lowers blood pressure (see Chapters 9 and 10).**

2. **Eliminate tobacco use, alcohol consumption, and excess caffeine (see Chapter 11).**

3. **Add a regular exercise regimen (see Chapter 12).**

Sometimes lifestyle modifications aren't enough to help lower your blood pressure. Many times, blood pressure medications are needed to help. Your health-care provider will talk with you about your options; I cover the medications used to treat high blood pressure in detail in Chapter 13.

Medications aren't *substitutes* for lifestyle changes — they're *additions* to lifestyle changes.

REMEMBER

Evaluating High Blood Pressure in Children, Women, and Older People

When evaluating and treating high blood pressure in children, pregnant women, and older people, some special factors come into play:

>> Older people usually have other complicating medical conditions, are taking other medications, and may have significant side effects from the medications they're taking. Turn to Chapter 15 for more on treating high blood pressure in people 65 and older.

>> More and more children and adolescents are being diagnosed with high blood pressure than ever before. I cover obesity and other factors related to high blood pressure in children in Chapter 16.

>> Throughout pregnancy, a woman is making new hormones while her body undergoes major changes. The high blood pressure that occasionally develops as a direct complication of pregnancy can harm both a mother and her unborn baby (see Chapter 17).

Chapter **2**

Detecting High Blood Pressure

If you've ever had your blood pressure measured during a typical visit to your doctor's office, it probably went something like this: You sat in the waiting room waiting for your appointment with your doctor. A nurse opened the door, called out your name, and hurriedly escorted you to the scale. You rushed to empty your pockets and take off your shoes before hopping on the scale. Then you were whisked back to the exam room and asked to sit on the exam table with your legs dangling. Your blood pressure was measured a couple minutes after you entered the exam room if not sooner. (Sometimes you can barely confirm your birth date before they have that blood pressure cuff around your arm.)

In this chapter, I explain why this approach isn't likely to give you a proper measurement of your blood pressure. To diagnose high blood pressure accurately, you need to have your blood pressure measured correctly. In this chapter, I explain how to take your blood pressure the right way. Whether you're taking your blood pressure at home or having it taken at your doctor's office, the treatment regimen begins with an accurate blood pressure reading.

In this chapter, I also explain what the numbers mean and the newest guidelines regarding high blood pressure.

Looking at the Gauge Used to Measure Blood Pressure

In the olden days, we used a blood pressure gauge called a *sphygmomanometer*. It consisted of a cuff that went around your arm above the elbow. The *bladder* was the part of the cuff that filled with air. A tube connected the cuff to a column of mercury (that looks like an outdoor thermometer) at one end and a rubber bulb at the other. When the rubber bulb was squeezed, the air pressure in this closed system forced the column of mercury to rise as the bladder filled with air. Numbers along the column of mercury indicated how much pressure is present.

For years, the mercury blood pressure gauge was considered the gold standard for blood pressure measurement. But that's not the case anymore. Today's aneroid blood pressure cuffs are portable, with a small blood pressure gauge and bulb (see Figure 2-1).

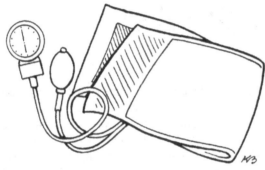

FIGURE 2-1:
An aneroid blood pressure gauge.

Illustration by Kathryn Born, MA

An alternative blood pressure measurement instrument that is commonly used in medical offices, as well as for home blood pressure monitoring, is the *oscillometric* or automated blood pressure gauge.

As technology has advanced, so have the devices used to measure blood pressure. You may encounter some medical offices that use manual blood pressure cuffs to measure blood pressure, but many health professionals are now using automated blood pressure machines instead.

WARNING

Don't rely on blood pressure measurements you can get in supermarkets or pharmacies. They may not give you an accurate reading.

THE WHITE-COAT EFFECT

The *white-coat effect* is elevated blood pressure that only happens in a doctor's office (many doctors wear white lab coats). For many people, something about being in a medical office and seeing the white coat causes their blood pressure to be elevated.

If your doctor initially gets a high reading, make sure they take it again at least five to ten minutes later. Your blood pressure may decrease during the visit.

People with white-coat high blood pressure are thought to be at an increased risk for developing cardiovascular disease compared to people with normal blood pressure. If you have white-coat high blood pressure, your doctor will want to figure out if it truly is just the white-coat effect, or if you have undiagnosed high blood pressure.

One way to get a definitive idea of whether you have high blood pressure is to have *ambulatory blood pressure monitoring* (see the "Getting an ambulatory reading" sidebar in this chapter). If the ambulatory monitoring shows high readings, your high blood pressure is real and should be treated accordingly.

Taking Your Blood Pressure Correctly

Unlike the typical scenario I describe at the beginning of this chapter, where you're rushed back to the exam room and you have your blood pressure taken almost immediately, a better scenario would go something like this: You sit in the waiting room waiting for your appointment with your doctor. A nurse opened the door, calls out your name, and escorts you to the scale and then to the exam room. You're asked to sit in a chair with your feet flat on the floor (without your legs crossed). You're told that your doctor will be with you in a few minutes, and you're asked to relax and breathe deeply until then. The nurse may even turn off the lights and close the door so you can focus on your breath.

Sound too good be true? Maybe, but the point is that you should be seated in a chair, feet flat on the ground, legs uncrossed. Your back should be straight, and you should be as relaxed. Your blood pressure shouldn't be taken as soon as you sit down.

Follow these few guidelines to get an accurate reading:

>> Don't smoke or drink alcohol or coffee within 30 minutes of a blood pressure measurement.

>> Sit with your back and arm supported. Your supported elbow should be at about the level of your heart.

>> Keep your feet on the ground.

>> Rest for several minutes in that position before the measurement.

>> Remain silent during the measurement.

TIP

When measuring blood pressure, it's a good idea to know what the reading is in both arms. When repeating future blood pressure measurements, use the arm that has the higher blood pressure reading.

WARNING

There should not be more than a 10- to 15-point difference between the blood pressures in both arms. If there is, your doctor may need to evaluate the arm with the lower blood pressure to make sure there is no narrowing or blockage of the blood flow in the arteries of that arm.

If you've been diagnosed with high blood pressure, you'll need to take your blood pressure at home on a regular basis. This is especially important if you're started a new blood pressure medication or if the dose or frequency of your medication has been changed. There are a number of advantages to measuring your own blood pressure at home:

>> Frequent measurements of your blood pressure can tell you whether your treatment is working, and you can track your blood pressure at different times of the day.

>> You can determine if your lifestyle changes (see Part 3) and/or medications are working. If they aren't, you can alter the treatment long before your next office visit by getting in touch with your doctor.

>> If your blood pressure remains steady and low, you may not have to see your doctor as frequently.

TIP

To use an automated blood pressure monitor at home, follow these steps:

1. **Sit in a chair with your back straight and your feet on the floor (without your legs crossed).**

2. **Place the cuff over your arm about 1 inch above the bend of your elbow.**

3. **Close the cuff around your arm, sticking the Velcro ends together at the end of the cuff.**

   If you have a large, muscular arm, that may cause an inaccurately high reading. Be sure to use a blood pressure gauge with a cuff that's large enough to accommodate your arm.

4. **Relax for about 5 minutes.**

5. **Place your arm at heart level (for example, lying straight out in front of you on a table or desk), and press the Start button on the machine.**

   You'll feel the cuff tighten around your arm, and then it will slowly loosen. It should beep or let you know when it's done. (Read the instructions of your particular device to find out exactly how it works.)

Many automated blood pressure machines have an automatic electronic memory built in that will keep a record of your blood pressures. Check the manual of your blood pressure device to see for how long a time it stores the blood pressure readings. You may want to keep your own record on paper or using an app on your phone.

TIP

If you're planning to buy an automated blood pressure cuff, make sure the device you buy is accurate. The American Medical Association has a website that lists devices that have been evaluated for accuracy. Just head to www.validatebp.org for more information.

REMEMBER

Studies have shown that people who measure their own blood pressure are more likely to stay on a regimen for lowering their blood pressure. Measuring your blood pressure at home is important!

GETTING AN AMBULATORY READING

Your doctor may want to check your blood pressure many times during one 24-hour period for a variety of reasons, including the following:

- To assess white-coat high blood pressure (see "The white-coat effect," earlier in this chapter)

- To determine whether you're resistant to medications and, if so, why

- To check low blood pressure symptoms

- To evaluate sporadic high blood pressure

Your doctor can't follow you around with a blood pressure gauge all day and night. So, they'll use a portable device called an *ambulatory blood pressure monitor*. This device consists of a cuff that attaches to your arm and to a machine. The machine pumps up the cuff and measures the blood pressure every 15 to 30 minutes during the day and every 30 to 60 minutes at night. The machine records the results and displays them when downloaded to a computer.

Understanding the Numbers

Over the years, different groups have established different goals for high blood pressure, and those goals have shifted as more research has been done. For example, the American Heart Association/American College of Cardiology (AHA/ACC) presented blood pressure guidelines in 2017 based on clinical studies (including the SPRINT trial, covered in Chapter 14). These new guidelines define high blood pressure as anything over 130/80 mm Hg. For this reason, most doctors aim for a blood pressure of 130/80 mm Hg in their patients, if not lower. But newer studies have demonstrated that a person with a blood pressure of 120/80 mm Hg is at lower risk of complications than a person with a blood pressure of 130/80 mm Hg or higher.

Table 2-1 shows the latest classifications of blood pressure for adults, according to the American Heart Association/American College of Cardiology. You can use this table to determine where your blood pressure falls (no pun intended) within these updated blood pressure guidelines. If your blood pressure falls in the elevated or high blood pressure categories, talk with your doctor about treatment options. *Note:* If your systolic blood pressure (SBP) and diastolic blood pressure (DBP) fall into two different categories, use the higher one. (Turn to the nearby sidebar, "Systolic and diastolic: The ups and downs of blood pressure," for more information.)

The goal with these new high blood pressure guidelines is to prevent complications from developing. The higher your blood pressure over time, the greater your risk for developing heart disease, kidney disease, and stroke.

TABLE 2-1   ## Classification of Blood Pressure for Adults

Category	SBP (in mm Hg)		DBP (in mm Hg)
Normal	Less than 120	and	Less than 80
Elevated blood pressure	120–129	and	Less than 80
High blood pressure, stage 1	130–139	or	80–89
High blood pressure, stage 2	140 or greater	or	90 or greater

TECHNICAL STUFF

SYSTOLIC AND DIASTOLIC: THE UPS AND DOWNS OF BLOOD PRESSURE

If your doctor says, "Your blood pressure is 135 over 85," what do those numbers really mean?

The first number is the *systolic blood pressure* (SBP), or the amount of pressure in your arteries as the heart pumps the blood to the rest of your body. *Systole* is the rhythmic contraction of your heart muscle when it's expelling blood from your left ventricle — the large chamber on the left side of your heart. The *aortic valve* sits between that chamber and your *aorta*, the large artery that takes blood away from the heart to the rest of the body. During systole, the aortic valve is open and blood flows freely to the rest of your body.

The second number is the *diastolic blood pressure* (DBP), the lowest point of blood pressure. After your heart empties the blood from the ventricle, the aortic valve shuts to prevent blood from returning into the heart from the rest of your body. Your heart muscle relaxes and the ventricle expands as blood from the lungs fills it up. At that moment, the blood pressure rapidly falls within your arteries until it reaches its DBP, its lowest point. Before the pressure falls further, the ventricle contracts again and the blood pressure starts to rise back up to the systolic level.

Lowering Blood Pressure Too Much

One common question about blood pressure is, "How low is too low?" Everyone has a different blood pressure they're able to tolerate. Your doctor's goal will be to lower your blood pressure to less than 130/80 mm Hg (or less than 120/80 mm Hg if possible), but you may not be able to tolerate a blood pressure this low. Signs that your blood pressure is too low includes dizziness and lightheadedness, especially when standing up.

WARNING

If your blood pressure has been high for years, it has caused changes in the blood vessels that can cause them to be more stiff, less pliable, and even narrowed. When you start taking a blood-pressure-lowering medication, you may not tolerate the decrease in blood pressure. The blood-pressure-lowering effect needs to take place over time to allow your body to adapt to the lower blood pressure.

A significant factor that can affect blood pressure outside of blood pressure medications is diabetes. Many people with diabetes can develop lowered blood pressure as they stand up, but have high blood pressure when standing or sitting. *Diabetic neuropathy* (nerve damage caused by diabetes) can affect how the body regulates blood pressure in different positions.

TIP

If you're started on a new blood pressure medication or you have diabetes, measure your blood pressure while you're in a standing position, especially if you're experiencing lightheadedness on standing. If a decrease of 20 mm Hg or more occurs in SBP or 10 mm Hg or more occurs in DBP, you have *orthostatic hypotension* (an abnormally great fall in blood pressure upon standing). If this occurs, talk with your doctor about adjusting your blood pressure medication.

Other things that may cause your blood pressure to get too low include:

>> Alcohol

>> Antidepressants

>> Anti-anxiety medications

>> Heart medications

>> Opiate pain medications

>> Medications used to treat an enlarged prostate

REMEMBER

Be sure to review all medications with your doctor.

In addition to diabetes, other medical conditions can affect blood pressure. Among them are

>> Changes in heart rhythm

>> Heart attack

>> Heart failure

>> Neurologic conditions in which blood pressure can be affected, such as Parkinson's disease

Getting the Right Assessment

When you're first diagnosed with high blood pressure, your doctor will have to make a number of assessments based on your medical history, a physical examination, and lab testing.

Reviewing your history

Your history describes your past experience with high blood pressure. It's similar to a history for any other condition, but it has a few variations specific to high blood pressure. The important points in the history are as follows:

>> Duration of high blood pressure (when it was first discovered)

>> Course of the blood pressure (whether it has always been high since it was discovered)

>> Prior treatment with medications, diet, exercise, or other means

>> Use of agents that can worsen blood pressure (such as steroids, birth control pills, and nonsteroidal anti-inflammatory drugs)

>> Use of over-the-counter medications such as decongestants or diet aids

>> Any family history of high blood pressure

>> Symptoms that may suggest resistant high blood pressure (see Chapter 4)

>> Symptoms of the consequences of high blood pressure (see Part 2)

>> Presence of other risk factors, like smoking, diabetes, high cholesterol, or kidney disease

>> Social factors like family structure, work, and education

>> Dietary history

>> Sexual function (certain blood pressure medications can affect it)

>> Possibility of *sleep apnea* (in which you gasp for breath and snore during sleep following several stops in breathing)

Having a physical exam

After your doctor talks to you about your history with high blood pressure, they'll do a physical exam. The main parts of the exam are as follows:

>> A blood pressure reading

>> An abdominal exam (to look for tumors or abnormal sounds suggesting restricted blood flow)

>> Evaluation of your body fat distribution and waist circumference (to look for *metabolic syndrome,* a condition often associated with high blood pressure in which you experience insulin resistance)

>> An examination of your neck (to look for thyroid or blood vessel abnormalities)

>> An examination of the pulses in the arteries (to look for evidence of peripheral vascular disease or decreased blood flow to your legs)

>> A heart exam (to look for any abnormal heart sounds or murmurs)

>> An internal eye exam (to look for signs of high blood pressure affecting the eyes)

>> A lung exam (to look for evidence of fluid in the lungs)

>> A neurological exam (to look for any areas of weakness or decreased strength)

Looking at lab tests

Your history and physical exam can give your doctor an excellent idea of the severity of the problem and the possibility that you have resistant high blood pressure (see Chapter 4). Lab tests provide a general picture of your overall health and look for specific abnormalities that the history and physical pointed to.

The key lab tests for everyone with high blood pressure are as follows:

>> Complete blood count (CBC)

>> Serum chemistry profile that looks at the sodium, potassium, glucose, liver function, and kidney function

>> Lipid profile that evaluates cholesterol and triglycerides

>> Microalbumin test to look for early kidney disease

Chapter **3**

Determining Whether You're at Risk

Many factors play a role in the development of high blood pressure. Some factors (such as your family history, ethnic background, age, and gender) you can't control. But others (such as nutrition, exercise, stress, and tobacco and alcohol use) you can control. These modifiable aspects are so important that I discuss them in detail in Part 3 of this book.

In this chapter, I fill you in on all the factors that can increase your risk of developing high blood pressure. If you haven't been diagnosed with high blood pressure, read up on the modifiable factors that can help reduce your risk of developing it. If you have been diagnosed with high blood pressure, be sure to read Part 3, where you can do a deep dive into things you can do to help lower your blood pressure, as well as improve your overall health.

Note: One thing that *can* cause your blood pressure to rise is forgetting your spouse's birthday. Running over your child's bike when you back into the garage is another. Fortunately, these elevations in blood pressure are only temporary!

TIP

Research regarding high blood pressure is ongoing. We're learning more and more about genetic and environmental aspects of high blood pressure. Check the appendix for references that provide all the latest and greatest news about this ever-evolving subject.

Reviewing Important Aspects of High Blood Pressure

This section describes the factors in your life that you can't control. You can't alter your family history, ethnic background, gender, and age. Although you can't control these risk factors, you still need to know how they contribute to high blood pressure, and you need to be cautious. Allow yourself to become obese, and you may have high blood pressure even though you're in a low-risk group.

TAKING A GLOBAL PERSPECTIVE

Worldwide, here's what high blood pressure looks like:

- Men have a slightly higher prevalence of high blood pressure than women, but approximately one-third of all men and women have high blood pressure.

- For men, the areas of the world with the highest occurrence of high blood pressure is in Eastern European and Central Asian countries; Southeast Asian countries have a very low occurrence of high blood pressure among men.

  For women, blood pressure is higher in the countries of Sub-Saharan Africa but lower in other areas of the world, including Latin America, Central Europe, and the Caribbean.

- In countries in which the population has a higher income, there is a decreased rate of high blood pressure compared to countries in which the population has a lower income.

For more information on social determinants of health — like access to healthy food, safe and affordable housing, and education and literacy — and its impact on health conditions including high blood pressure, visit https://health.gov/healthypeople/priority-areas/social-determinants-health.

Understanding the effect of genetics

REMEMBER

High blood pressure tends to run in families, so a family history of the condition can predict its development in relatives who have normal blood pressure. For example, when comparing biological children with adopted children, the same or similar blood pressure measurements were shared between biological parents and their children to a greater degree than between adopted children and their parents. Bottom line? If you have two or more relatives who developed high blood pressure before the age of 55, you're at much higher risk of developing it yourself. (Next time around, try to pick your parents a little more carefully!)

Multiple genes and proteins are involved in the genetics of high blood pressure. If you've been diagnosed with high blood pressure, especially if you were first diagnosed with high blood pressure by the time you were a young adult, your family history is important. Your doctor will want to discuss the following with you:

>> Has anyone else in your family been diagnosed with high blood pressure? If so, were they on your mother's side of the family or your father's side, or both?

>> Do any of your first-degree relatives (mother, father, sibling, children) have high blood pressure?

>> Is there any family history of kidney disease? If so, at what age was kidney disease first diagnosed?

>> Do any conditions run in your family? Examples include polycystic kidney disease or vascular disease affecting multiple blood vessels.

>> Do multiple people in your family ever have symptoms such as episodic dizziness, lightheadedness when standing up, palpitations, flushing, or episodic headaches?

TIP

Genetic testing is available for certain conditions related to high blood pressure; these conditions are usually affected by one gene that is causing the high blood pressure. If your health-care provider suspects a possible familial condition, they may want you to go for genetic testing.

Estimating the effects of ethnicity

According to the U.S. Centers for Disease Control and Prevention (CDC), the prevalence of high blood pressure is higher among men than women. Among men, the prevalence of high blood pressure among African-American males is higher

(57 percent) compared to Hispanic males (50 percent) and Caucasian males (50 percent). For women, the occurrence of high blood pressure was higher among African-American females (56 percent) compared to Hispanic females (36 percent) and Caucasian females (36 percent).

Seeing how medication can affect blood pressure

Medications that you're taking over the counter or by prescription can have an effect on your blood pressure. Here are a few examples:

» **Nonsteroidal anti-inflammatory drugs (NSAIDS):** Examples include ibuprofen and aspirin, among others. These drugs are commonly used by millions of people to treat pain. Side effects can include an increase in blood pressure and salt and water retention. NSAIDs also can blunt the blood-pressure-lowering effects of a class of blood-pressure-lowering medications called *diuretics* (see Chapter 13).

» **Oral contraceptives:** These medications can raise blood pressure. If you're taking oral contraceptives, your doctor will want to keep an eye on your blood pressure.

» **Certain chemotherapy medications:** Some commonly prescribed medications used in the treatment of cancer (for example, multikinase inhibitors) can cause high blood pressure. Before starting any chemotherapy, discuss the potential side effects with your health-care provider.

» **Antidepressants:** Medications used to treat depression can also raise blood pressure. One example is venlafaxine.

TIP

Talk with your health-care provider about any medications you're taking and whether they may put you at risk for developing high blood pressure.

Changing Your Lifestyle to Prevent High Blood Pressure

There are things you can do to improve your high blood pressure or even prevent high blood pressure from occurring. This topic is so important that Part 3 of this book is dedicated to it. For now, some examples of things you can do include the following:

>> Follow a healthy nutrition plan that's low in sodium and/or primarily plant based. Check out *DASH Diet For Dummies* by Sarah Samaan, Rosanne Rust, and Cindy Kleckner (Wiley) for guidelines and recipes.

>> Reduce your daily sodium intake to 2,400 mg (see Chapter 10).

>> Stop smoking and limit your alcohol consumption (see Chapter 11).

>> Follow an exercise plan (see Chapter 12).

>> Incorporate meditation, yoga, and/or deep meditative breathing into your daily routine (see Chapter 12).

REMEMBER

All the techniques that *prevent* high blood pressure can also help *lower* blood pressure after it's present. If you can prevent high blood pressure, do everything in your power to do so. Your body will thank you for it!

Chapter **4**

Reviewing the Causes of Resistant High Blood Pressure

Resistant high blood pressure (also referred to as *secondary high blood pressure*) is blood pressure that's difficult to control with medication.

TECHNICAL STUFF

Doctors use specific criteria to diagnose resistant high blood pressure. You have resistant high blood pressure if either of the following applies:

» You're taking three or more blood pressure medications (including a class of blood pressure medications called *diuretics*).

» You're taking four or more blood pressure medications at one time (and one of them is *not* a diuretic).

When doctors are looking for resistant causes of high blood pressure, they're looking for many of the specific conditions covered in this chapter. In many cases, treatment of the underlying condition improves or sometimes even eliminates the high blood pressure.

Resistant high blood pressure makes up only 8 percent to 10 percent of the total number of high blood pressure cases, but its causes are important. A careful history, physical exam, and lab evaluation can help your doctor discover possible medical conditions that are causing your blood pressure to rise and be resistant to medical treatment. This chapter introduces you to some of the most common causes of resistant high blood pressure, the way the diagnosis is confirmed in each case, and the appropriate treatment.

REMEMBER

If you've been diagnosed with resistant high blood pressure, the longer you've had the underlying condition, the more difficult it is to completely normalize the blood pressure despite treating that underlying condition. This is because no matter the cause, the blood vessels in your body become used to the effects of the high blood pressure. That said, many times resistant blood pressure *does* improve and you may be able to reduce the dosage or discontinue many of the blood pressure medications you're taking.

WARNING

Don't stop or reduce the dosage of any of your blood pressure medications without speaking to your doctor first. Some medications can't be stopped cold turkey but need to be reduced gradually because they can cause withdrawal symptoms.

Identifying the Signs and Symptoms of Resistant High Blood Pressure

In addition to high blood pressure that is resistant to medication (see the chapter intro for the technical definition of resistant high blood pressure), there are other clues you need to be aware of that should prompt your doctor to evaluate what's causing your resistant high blood pressure. These clues include the following:

>> Evidence of the heart, kidneys, or eyes being affected by high blood pressure (see Part 2 of this book for more information)

>> A family history of kidney disease or a history of high blood pressure in family members at a young age (for example, as children, teenagers, or even in their early 20s or 30s)

>> *Flushing spells* (in which you feel like your face is flushed and your skin turns red and hot) that come out of nowhere and resolve

- >> *Palpitations* (in which you feel your heart racing and/or notice that your pulse is fast) that occur independently and/or with other symptoms, including facial flushing, dizziness, or diarrhea

- >> Increased stretch marks over the abdomen and/or increased weight gain

- >> Intolerance to heat or cold

- >> Dizziness when standing up

- >> *Bruit* (a loud humming sound in the abdomen or lateral low back area) heard by a health-care provider with a stethoscope

- >> Low potassium level in the blood that never seems to get to a normal range despite taking a potassium supplement

- >> Rapid pulse with or without palpitations

- >> New onset of high blood pressure before age 20 or over the age of 50

- >> Unusually high blood pressure (above 180/120) when your blood pressure has previously been under control

If you experience any of these symptoms, make an appointment with your health-care provider — and don't wait. The sooner you treat resistant high blood pressure, the better.

REMEMBER

In trying to evaluate what's causing your blood pressure to be very difficult to treat, your doctor will likely ask you lots of questions about the symptoms listed earlier, among other things. You may have more than one of these symptoms, and sometimes the totality of the symptoms together can help your doctor home in on a possible diagnosis. The other reason your doctor may give you the third degree is that some symptoms can overlap with multiple conditions — for example, palpitations and flushing can be noted in a few causes of resistant high blood pressure. Being thorough is really important in getting to the bottom of what's keeping your blood pressure elevated.

Considering Chronic Kidney Disease and High Blood Pressure

If you've had resistant high blood pressure, one important consideration is chronic kidney disease (CKD). Chapter 6 covers the kidneys in depth, but I'm mentioning CKD here because it's the most common cause of resistant high blood pressure.

CKD is defined as abnormal kidney function, as detected on a blood test that your doctor can order, that lasts at least three months. If a blood test shows abnormal kidney function, your doctor will want you to be retested every few months to make the diagnosis. In many cases, CKD is undiagnosed, especially if the person feels well and has no symptoms.

High blood pressure in and of itself is a major cause of CKD, and CKD (no matter the cause) can cause high blood pressure that can, over time, be resistant to treatment.

There are many causes of CKD. High blood pressure and diabetes are the two leading causes — in fact, many times, they occur together. Other conditions that affect the kidneys can include conditions that block the flow of urine, certain medications, inflammatory processes, and/or inherited conditions. Regardless of the cause, the first step is diagnosing that CKD is present in the first place. From there, your doctor will do more testing and/or ask a *nephrologist* (kidney specialist) to do more testing to figure out what's causing your CKD.

Blood pressure control is important in CKD because it can further affect the kidneys and lead to even higher blood pressure. The treatment for CKD is focused on identifying the cause of CKD and treating the cause.

Navigating Narrowed Renal Arteries

Certain conditions can cause blockage to the blood flow of the kidneys, resulting in what's known as *renal vascular hypertension.* (*Renal* refer to the kidneys, *vascular* refers to the blood vessels, and *hypertension* is the technical name for high blood pressure.) The aorta is like a large tree trunk with branches that provide blood flow to the various organs of the body. The main blood flow to each kidney comes from one branch off the aorta.

Conditions that cause renal vascular hypertension block one or both kidney arteries (a condition known as *renal artery stenosis*). When the obstruction keeps a kidney from receiving enough blood flow, the kidney produces a hormone called *renin.* The kidney knows it isn't getting the blood flow it needs, but it doesn't know why. You can think of renin as a "kidney defense mechanism." Renin acts on other hormones to try to raise the blood pressure and maintain the blood flow to the kidney. Because the original obstruction keeps the increased blood pressure from delivering more blood to the kidney, the high blood pressure continues.

Diagnosing renal artery stenosis

Certain conditions can cause renal artery stenosis (RAS), or the obstruction of one or both of the kidney arteries. These conditions include the following:

>> **Atherosclerotic renal artery stenosis (ARAS):** This condition occurs in older people, most commonly in the early part of the renal artery or right at the branch point of the renal artery off of the aorta. In this process, cholesterol plaque is deposited in the arteries, eventually causing the arteries to narrow. ARAS usually occurs in middle-aged and older men and women, and it accounts for two-thirds of all causes of blocked kidney arteries. Often, vascular disease is found elsewhere in the body — for example, someone with ARAS may also have heart disease, carotid artery disease, and/or peripheral vascular disease (PVD).

>> **Fibromuscular dysplasia (FMD):** Instead of being caused by deposits of plaque in the artery, fibromuscular dysplasia (FMD) is caused by a thickening of the muscle in the artery. This condition is seen in younger people, especially in teenagers. FMD tends to occur in the latter or distal part of the renal artery. The most common presentation of this is new-onset high blood pressure in a young person. In a small percentage of people, the carotid arteries can also be affected by FMD.

Other conditions may affect the blood flow to the kidneys, but these two are most commonly seen.

TIP

Why would a doctor suspect that ARAS may be the cause of your resistant high blood pressure? In addition to signs and symptoms listed earlier in the chapter, the following symptoms indicate that ARAS may be present:

>> **Vascular disease (especially PVD) elsewhere in the body:** Vascular disease increases the risk of ARAS being present. This risk is really heightened if there is a history of high blood pressure, diabetes, and smoking.

>> **Recurrent congestive heart failure in the absence of any significant cardiac abnormalities or valvular disease:** This is a unique presentation of ARAS in older individuals.

>> **Bruit:** Bruit can signal common causes of RAS, but it can be heard in only 50 percent of cases.

TECHNICAL
STUFF

FMD is more commonly seen in younger people — teenagers or young adults with a new onset of high blood pressure. They're less likely to present with significant peripheral vascular disease or recurrent congestive heart failure (symptoms that usually occur in older adults).

TECHNICAL STUFF

Sometimes a low potassium level can be seen in the blood with RAS due to either ARAS or FMD. This is because, when the blood flow to a kidney is blocked, that kidney is making a lot of the hormone renin, which causes the formation of other hormones, including aldosterone, which can cause the low potassium levels.

If your doctor suspects RAS, they can order some specific testing to further evaluate. Here are a couple tests you may come across if you're being evaluated for this condition:

>> **Renal artery Doppler ultrasound:** A renal ultrasound looks at the blood flow to the kidneys and is used to determine if there is a narrowing of the arteries. An advantage of this test is that it doesn't require the use of any *intravenous contrast* (where they inject a dye into your blood), which can affect kidney function. The disadvantage is that it can't pinpoint exactly *where* the blockage is. But it's a good initial study.

TIP

If you're ever scheduled for an ultrasound test with the word *Doppler* in it, the test is looking at the blood flow of that particular vascular structure or organ. For example, lower extremity arterial Doppler looks at the arterial blood flow to the legs to see if there is a blockage present. A carotid Doppler looks at the blood flow to the carotid arteries in the neck to see if there is a blockage of blood flow.

>> **Computed tomography (CT) angiogram:** This special kind of CT scan uses dye and is a noninvasive test to help determine the area that is blocked. It's a diagnostic study that can tell if there is a narrowing in the arteries to your kidneys.

There is a minor risk of dye exposure with this test. In some individuals, especially if they're dehydrated, the dye can worsen the kidney function. Your doctor will discuss this testing with you, as well as ways to minimize the dye risk to the kidneys (including making sure you're properly hydrated before the test and temporarily holding some medications the day of the test).

Treating blocked renal arteries

Treatment of blocked renal arteries depends on the cause.

If you have FMD, this condition is very much amenable to angioplasty. FMD is due to a very thickened muscular area in the blood vessel, not plaque deposits. During angioplasty, the surgeon inserts a *catheter* (a slender, hollow tube) into the artery and widens the artery with a balloon.

For ARAS, medical therapy with blood pressure control, statins, stopping smoking, and lifestyle modifications are just as effective as intervention to open up a blocked renal artery.

However, there are times when intervention for ARAS is indicated:

>> When blood pressure is dangerously high (for example, over 180/100) despite being on multiple medications and the risk of stroke or bleeding is significant because of uncontrolled blood pressure

>> When the kidneys are drastically affected by RAS such that the kidney function is really, really compromised and, without any intervention to open up the blockage, the kidney function will get worse and the person will end up needing dialysis

>> When someone has recurrent episodes of heart failure and the heart is otherwise normal

These three situations are extreme and somewhat uncommon. The more common situation is one where there is a blockage but the kidney function is stable and blood pressure is controlled on three or more medications. There is no advantage in that situation for an intervention. Why? Because an angioplasty or placement of a stent isn't without risk.

WARNING

There are some issues with regards to angioplasty and stent as they relate to ARAS:

>> **Medical therapy with drugs is highly effective for many years in more than half of patients.**

>> **Angioplasty fails to lower blood pressure in up to 40 percent of patients.** If you've had high blood pressure for years, the artery itself changes — it becomes more thickened, scarred, and less pliable — and it's less likely that an angioplasty and stent would help to improve your blood pressure.

>> **Kidney function worsens in at least 20 percent of patients treated with angioplasty.** This worsening is due to the dye used or to a complication of the procedure, or a combination of both.

>> **The disease recurs in up to 5 percent to 10 percent of patients who are initially successful, although the use of a specialized stent decreases this risk.**

WARNING

If someone has bilateral ARAS, the use of a class of medications called angiotensin-converting enzyme (ACE) inhibitors can make the kidney function worse because of their effect on certain renal hormones including renin in this situation. If someone is started on this medication and repeat blood work shows significant worsening of kidney function (as well as a significant lowering of blood pressure in some individuals), this is another sign that ARAS may be present and affecting both kidneys.

Homing in on Hormones That Cause Hypertension

Some organs make *hormones* (chemical messengers that trigger chemical reactions or the production of other proteins or hormones), but sometimes an organ can make too *much* of a certain hormone. Other times, there can be something else in the body (an *adenoma*, or benign mass) that can produce too much of a hormone. Hormones can elevate blood pressure to an abnormal extent.

Adenomas usually originate in an *adrenal gland* (one adrenal gland sits on top of each of your kidneys; see Figure 4-1), but they can also sometimes be seen in other parts of the body, including in nerve tissues. The adrenal glands secrete the following hormones:

>> **Epinephrine:** This hormone usually helps to maintain normal blood pressure and blood glucose. In excess, it can raise blood pressure and cause a rapid heart rate.

>> **Aldosterone:** This hormone helps to regulate blood pressure and salt and water levels in the bloodstream. When made in excess, aldosterone can raise blood pressure and lower potassium levels in some people.

>> **Cortisol:** This hormone helps to regulate blood glucose levels and plays a role in maintaining blood pressure. In excess, it can raise both glucose levels and blood pressure.

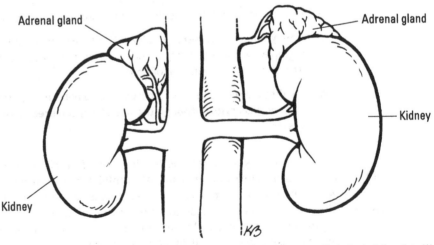

Adrenal gland

Adrenal gland

Kidney

FIGURE 4-1:
Your adrenal glands are on top of your kidneys.

Kidney

Illustration by Kathryn Born, MA

Figure 4-2 shows the different parts of the adrenal gland and the part responsible for the various hormones described in this section.

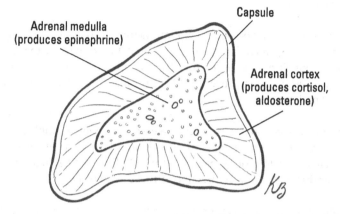

Adrenal medulla
(produces epinephrine)

Capsule

Adrenal cortex
(produces cortisol,
aldosterone)

Illustration by Kathryn Born, MA

FIGURE 4-2:
The parts of the
adrenal gland
and its
hormones.

Finding an epinephrine-producing tumor

Epinephrine and norepinephrine, normal products of the adrenal gland, raise blood pressure, heart rate, and blood glucose during stressful times and cause sweating as well. Sometimes a *pheochromocytoma* (a tumor that releases large quantities of norepinephrine) can arise in an adrenal gland (shown with the kidneys in Figure 4-1) or may be found along the nerve tissues of the body.

A pheochromocytoma is rare (occurring in only 6 out of 100,000 people who have high blood pressure), but the symptoms often can occur suddenly, especially in response to a stressful event. It often occurs spontaneously, with an acute rise in blood pressure due to a sudden release of norepinephrine. The sudden release of a large amount of norepinephrine can have dire consequences if it isn't diagnosed and treated.

WARNING

The most common symptoms of a pheochromocytoma include the following:

>> Headache

>> Palpitations

>> *Tachycardia* (rapid heart rate)

>> Excessive sweating

>> Dizziness when standing up

If high blood pressure is present but you feel none of these symptoms, the diagnosis of a pheochromocytoma is extremely unlikely. High blood pressure is sustained in more than half of patients with pheochromocytoma, but it may be intermittent.

Significant stressors can precipitate acute episode of palpitations, tachycardia, and sweating, including but not limited to exercise, urination, defecation, an enema, smoking, examination of the abdomen, and anesthesia. The symptoms can vary from mild to severe, and the timing of the symptoms can be different for every patient.

WARNING

Certain cheeses (including aged cheddar) and many alcohol-containing beverages (including beer and wine) contain a chemical called *tyramine,* which may bring on a headache, palpitations, and sweating. Medications like histamine, glucagon, and phenothiazines can also precipitate these symptoms.

REMEMBER

A pheochromocytoma is suspected much more often than it actually occurs simply because its symptoms are the same as those of a healthy person who is nervous and upset. The symptoms can mimic a panic attack; the palpitations, fast heart rate, and sweating can mimic some other causes of resistant high blood pressure, too.

The following steps explain how your doctor will diagnose this uncommon condition:

1. **They'll order a blood test for plasma *metanephrines* (a breakdown product of epinephrine).**

   Breakdown products result when epinephrine is converted to an inactive form in the body. Blood testing is done first, before any imaging studies are ordered.

2. **If your metanephrine level is elevated, your doctor will ask you to collect urine for 24 hours.**

   This test checks for the presence of metanephrines and *normetanephrines* (other breakdown products of epinephrine).

3. **If elevated levels of metanephrine are found, your doctor will want to use specialized imaging procedures, including a CT scan or *magnetic resonance imaging* (MRI) scan to look for a mass producing these hormones.**

   Most pheochromocytomas are located in the adrenal gland, but 15 percent of them arise in another location, such as the nerve tissue, the abdomen, or the chest cavity. (If the tumor is in one of these locations and is more than 2 centimeters in size, the scan can see it there as well.) A surgeon may have to find the tumor during surgery; usually, surgeons look for more than one tumor. About 10 percent of pheochromocytomas are malignant.

4. **If needed, other specialized imaging procedures can be done; these are often ordered by a nephrologist or *endocrinologist* (a doctor specializing in the endocrine glands).**

Some forms of pheochromocytomas run in families as solitary pheochromocytomas or with other associated conditions. When several different types of tumors are present, the condition is referred to as *multiple endocrine neoplasia* (MEN) and can involve other glands. Your health-care provider will ask you questions about your family history and also examine the functioning of other organs, including the thyroid and parathyroid glands. Your doctor should look for tumors of the thyroid and parathyroid glands whenever a pheochromocytoma and MEN are suspected.

TIP

These cases are extremely rare. If your doctor thinks you might have this condition, you may be referred to a specialist at a major academic center who sees more patients with this condition.

Treating a pheochromocytoma

Surgery removes most pheochromocytomas, but first your blood pressure has to be under control. Your doctor may prescribe phenoxybenzamine or doxazosin to block the action of epinephrine and control your high blood pressure. You need to be on this medication for approximately one week; this is often enough to help control your blood pressure before surgery and prevent the sudden release of norepinephrine either during anesthesia or during the surgery itself.

WARNING

If your blood pressure isn't controlled before surgery, the mortality rate can be really high. The chances of the blood pressure *not* being controlled before surgery are extremely slim.

The surgery to remove the mass is laparoscopic, done through a small incision in the abdomen. A tube is inserted, and the tumor is localized and removed. Given the rarity of this condition, the surgery is more commonly performed at major academic centers.

As with other causes of resistant high blood pressure, the high blood pressure may persist after surgery if you've had this condition for years before diagnosis. If so, you'll need blood pressure medication.

Detecting a tumor that produces aldosterone

There are three layers of the adrenal gland, and each layer is responsible for the production of certain hormones. The *adrenal cortex* (the outer covering of the adrenal gland; refer to Figure 4-2) produces aldosterone, an important hormone that's responsible for regulating blood pressure, maintaining sodium balance, and eliminating potassium from the body. *Primary hyperaldosteronism* (either due to the adrenal glands themselves making a lot of aldosterone or due to aldosterone-producing tumor in one of the adrenal glands) causes an overabundance of aldosterone to be produced — much more than the human body needs. The large amount of aldosterone causes significant sodium retention, potassium loss (about 50 percent of the time), and high blood pressure.

The number of individuals diagnosed with this condition is thought to be underestimated; primary hyperaldosteronism may, in fact, represent up to 20 percent to 25 percent of all cases of resistant high blood pressure. Many times, the cause of resistant high blood pressure may not be found despite a detailed diagnostic evaluation. These cases are often diagnosed as *idiopathic* (fancy medical jargon meaning "we don't know what's causing it"). It seems that a fair number of these cases of resistant high blood pressure may be due to primary hyperaldosteronism.

The following caveats are important to keep in mind with primary hyperaldosteronism:

» As many as one in ten people with high blood pressure may have primary hyperaldosteronism (not necessarily due to a mass on the adrenal gland producing aldosterone).

» Primary hyperaldosteronism should be considered in every case of high blood pressure, even when the potassium is normal. The potassium level can be normal 50 percent of the time — low potassium level does *not* rule out this condition.

» Blood tests should determine the ratio of aldosterone and renin levels in the bloodstream. With this condition, blood testing is needed first to make the diagnosis before imaging studies are ordered.

Diagnosing primary hyperaldosteronism

The two main causes of primary hyperaldosteronism are aldosterone-producing adenoma and hyperplasia of both adrenal glands (in which the portion of the adrenal glands that make aldosterone gets bigger and makes more aldosterone).

The first step to diagnose this condition is checking the blood aldosterone and renin levels. In primary hyperaldosteronism, the aldosterone levels are high and the renin levels in the blood are very low to undetectable. The classic teaching regarding this condition has been: If the ratio of high aldosterone and low renin is not found, it isn't primary hyperaldosteronism.

However, there is a significant nuance regarding this condition that changes the whole way that health-care providers are now thinking about it: The aldosterone level is not always high and renin level is not always low at the time of testing. This idea is relatively new regarding this condition and may help explain why the condition is underdiagnosed.

Think of it this way: We initially thought of aldosterone as a hormone that was continually produced either from hyperplasia or from an adenoma in which the renin is suppressed 24/7. But this isn't the case. Aldosterone is a hormone, and its production can vary throughout the day, even in primary hyperaldosteronism. This means that depending on when an aldosterone or renin level is obtained, the results may vary and the test may not always show an elevated aldosterone and low renin level.

TIP

If you're diagnosed with resistant high blood pressure and an initial renin and aldosterone test shows that you don't have primary hyperaldosteronism, the renin and aldosterone levels may need to be repeated a couple more times at different times of the day to really rule out the diagnosis.

Your health-care provider may order other sophisticated tests to confirm this diagnosis, but the take-home point is this: If you're diagnosed with resistant high blood pressure, talk to your doctor about primary hyperaldosteronism and the need for multiple testing results.

Other clues to this condition can include the following:

>> High blood pressure (may be as high as over 180/110).

>> Increased potassium in the urine and low potassium levels in the blood. If the potassium levels in the blood are really low, you may have significant muscle weakness. (Again, the potassium may be low in the blood less than 50 percent of the time, so a normal potassium level doesn't rule out primary hyperaldosteronism.)

>> Increased sodium levels in the blood.

Because the blood pressure can be so high, individuals with primary hyperaldosteronism are at increased risk of an acute stroke, CKD due to undiagnosed or resistant high blood pressure, hypertensive heart disease, and damage to the kidneys (see Part 2 for more about these consequences of high blood pressure).

REMEMBER

Normally, renin is produced by the kidneys, which leads to the production of aldosterone by the adrenal gland. With primary hyperaldosteronism, the renin level is low — a sign that an aldosterone-producing process (either an adenoma or hyperplasia, and not renin) is stimulating the production of aldosterone.

In RAS, a kidney with insufficient blood pressure produces renin. This renin causes the production of *angiotensin II* (a strong blood-vessel constriction agent that also triggers the release of aldosterone) from angiotensin I (another blood pressure–type hormone). In this situation, renin is elevated (not suppressed), which stimulates aldosterone.

After biochemical testing (repeated testing showing high aldosterone and low/suppressed renin levels) are present, the diagnosis is either an aldosterone-secreting adenoma or *bilateral adrenal hyperplasia* (increased aldosterone production in both adrenal glands). This distinction is important because bilateral adrenal hyperplasia tends to be a milder disease than an aldosterone-producing adenoma, and it doesn't respond well to surgery. In order to figure this out, imaging studies are needed.

A CT or MRI scan of the abdomen can often distinguish a solitary adrenal adenoma from bilateral hyperplasia. Sometimes the scan doesn't make the distinction because aldosterone-producing tumors tend to be small and the incidence of *incidentalomas* (nonfunctional growths) on the adrenal gland is high. In that case, an interventional radiologist does a specialized procedure, placing a tube into the adrenal veins on each side of the body and looking for large amounts of aldosterone in the sample.

If one side has a lot of aldosterone and the other side doesn't, the diagnosis is an aldosterone-producing adenoma, not bilateral hyperplasia. Specialized testing is used to make the diagnosis.

LOVING LICORICE CAN LOWER YOUR RENIN

Believe it or not, eating lots of licorice can raise your blood pressure and lower the amount of renin in your bloodstream. A steady consumption of licorice can block the enzyme that normally converts cortisol (which maintains blood glucose and helps maintain blood pressure) to cortisone (an anti-inflammatory hormone) in the kidney. Because cortisol has some activity similar to aldosterone in test results and cortisone doesn't, the unusually high concentrations of cortisol *clinically* imitates increased levels of aldosterone in the body. But a more accurate picture can be drawn from a patient's history of licorice eating and their low aldosterone test results. It usually requires four weeks of eating anywhere from one to five sticks (50 to 100 grams) of licorice every day for this effect to occur.

Treating primary hyperaldosteronism

The treatment of a solitary adrenal adenoma that makes too much aldosterone is laparoscopic surgery to remove the tumor. Before surgery, the doctor prescribes *spironolactone*, a drug that reverses the action of aldosterone, for several days.

After surgery, the aldosterone level falls, the potassium returns to normal, and the blood pressure returns to normal. Sometimes the blood pressure stays up because you also have *essential high blood pressure* (high blood pressure for which the cause can't be determined) or because permanent damage has taken place in the blood vessels or kidneys. This problem occurs most often with individuals who've had high blood pressure for several years.

Sometimes people aren't candidates for surgery or may not want to undergo surgery. Medical treatment with medications that block aldosterone (the most commonly prescribed medication being spironolactone) is often successful. Spironolactone does have significant side effects, including breast enlargement with nipple tenderness and a decreased interest in sex for some individuals. Discuss these potential side effects with your doctor before taking this medication.

If the cause of primary hyperaldosteronism is bilateral adrenal hyperplasia, your doctor will treat it medically with spironolactone. Removal of the adrenal glands doesn't generally cure the high blood pressure even though the low potassium improves.

TIP

Another medication in the same class as spironolactone, is an option for bilateral adrenal hyperplasia and adrenal adenomas because it reverses the low potassium (if present) and the high blood pressure without causing the sexual side effects of spironolactone.

Recognizing Cushing's syndrome

In addition to pheochromocytoma and primary aldosteronism, the adrenal gland can be the site of yet another resistant high blood pressure source, *Cushing's syndrome*, in which the adrenal glands make too much cortisol. Cushing's syndrome can present in three different ways:

>> **Most of the time, an excessive production of *adrenocorticotrophin* (ACTH, the pituitary hormone that regulates the adrenal gland) caused by a tumor in the pituitary, stimulates both adrenal glands to make too much cortisol.** If a tumor forms in the pituitary gland, it can cause the adrenal glands to make too much cortisol and other steroids that have plenty of salt-retaining activity. As a result, the blood pressure rises.

>> **In the remaining cases, there is a tumor in one of the adrenal glands.** When the adrenal tumor makes too much cortisol independently of ACTH, the ACTH is suppressed instead of elevated.

>> **In less than 2 percent of cases, an adrenal-stimulating hormone from some other tumor in the body (particularly a lung cancer) stimulates the adrenal glands.** This condition is *ectopic* (from an abnormal site) ACTH production. The result is Cushing's syndrome, but it tends to be more aggressive, producing low potassium levels. The ectopic source often has some identifying symptom such as cough from a lung cancer.

Diagnosing Cushing's syndrome

Cushing's syndrome is associated with high blood pressure that's difficult to treat. It may be as high as 180/110, if not higher. The syndrome occurs three times more often in women than in men and often in a person's 30s or 40s. The mortality rate from untreated Cushing's syndrome is high, approximately 10 percent.

Too much cortisol in the bloodstream has other properties that can manifest as:

>> High blood glucose levels and the development of diabetes

>> Easy bruising of the body

>> Loss of bone with development of osteoporosis, which causes spontaneous fractures

>> Obesity of the trunk of the body with thin arms and legs

>> Psychological changes ranging from irritability and agitation to severe depression

>> Purplish stretch marks, especially on the abdomen

In addition to high blood pressure, depending on the cause of Cushing's syndrome, other possible symptoms include

>> Headache caused by the pituitary tumor

>> Pigmentation of certain areas of the body

>> Loss of menstrual function in women due to the adrenal glands producing excessive amounts of hormones that have masculinizing properties

>> Hairiness in women due to the same masculinizing hormones

Given all these signs and symptoms, Cushing's syndrome is relatively easy to prove with blood tests. Often two different tests are used to confirm the diagnosis before any imaging studies are obtained. The first test is called a low-dose dexamethasone test, in which a person takes 1 mg of *dexamethasone* (a steroid hormone much like cortisol) at midnight. The next morning, a blood test is done to check the cortisol level.

If 1 mg of dexamethasone decreases cortisol production, then Cushing's syndrome is *not* present. If the cortisol is appropriately suppressed, no further testing is needed. If the cortisol level is elevated, a 24-hour urine collection is tested; a high amount of cortisol in the urine indicates that Cushing's syndrome is present. A salivary cortisol test can also be used in place of the urine test.

When the screening test is positive, a blood test measures the amount of ACTH in the bloodstream. ACTH is a hormone made by the pituitary normally to stimulate cortisol production. If the cortisol level is high, part of the diagnostic evaluation is to see if the ACTH levels are high or low.

Imaging studies are also needed in the diagnostic evaluation. For example, an MRI of the brain may be ordered to evaluate the pituitary gland. Other imaging tests include a CT scan or MRI of the abdomen to look at the adrenal glands.

REMEMBER

Blood tests are the first step to make the diagnosis. Imaging studies are used only after the blood testing confirms the diagnosis. The blood tests also enable your health-care provider to determine which imaging studies are the most appropriate.

Treating Cushing's syndrome

The first step in treating Cushing's syndrome is to control the blood pressure with medication. The choices are the same as for essential high blood pressure (see Chapter 13). After the blood pressure is under control, the treatment is directed to the source of the excess hormone:

>> If the pituitary gland is responsible through an ACTH-producing lesion, surgery or another interventional procedure may be required. If an adrenal gland has a mass causing increased cortisol production, surgery is indicated to remove the mass.

WARNING

>> If surgery is performed on the pituitary or the adrenal glands, steroid replacement may be needed to provide the cortisol that your body isn't able to produce because of the surgical procedure. Steroids are essential to life, so this is something your health-care team will discuss with you if surgery is needed.

Evaluating Other Causes of Resistant High Blood Pressure

There are a few other treatable conditions associated with high blood pressure. Most of them are reversible, and the high blood pressure responds to the correction of the disease unless it has been present for some time.

Coarctation of the aorta

Coarctation of the aorta is a narrowing of the large artery that leaves the heart. Depending on the severity, the narrowing is usually present at birth though not diagnosed until the teenage or early adult years. The narrowing is usually close to the beginning of the aorta but below where the artery branches to the arms. The result is high blood pressure in the arms and lower blood pressure in the legs (which the doctor can observe by simply measuring the blood pressure in the arms and legs).

The narrowing results in the production of a *murmur* (a humming sound), which your doctor can hear with a stethoscope in the area of the heart. In addition, your doctor won't be able to detect a pulse in the groin. The kidneys respond to the lower blood pressure by putting out more renin; the increase leads to even higher blood pressure above the narrowing but not below it.

Children with this condition can have nosebleeds, dizziness, pounding headaches, and, when they exercise, leg cramps.

During a careful first examination of any baby, the doctor feels for the pulses in the feet and notes whether pulses are present. If they aren't, the doctor can order further evaluation with a CT scan or MRI of the chest.

The treatment consists of surgery to open the narrow area or sometimes *balloon angioplasty*, the same technique used to open the narrow blood vessels of the heart. (See the "Treating blocked renal arteries" section, earlier in this chapter for more on angioplasty.)

WARNING

If the coarctation isn't treated, the patient may die before the age of 40 from complications of high blood pressure.

Too much or too little thyroid hormone

Both *hyperthyroidism* (too much thyroid hormone) and *hypothyroidism* (too little thyroid hormone) can be associated with high blood pressure. These conditions may be easy to diagnose if the symptoms are significant, but hypothyroidism is often subtle.

>> If the patient has a rapid pulse, weight loss, and sweating in addition to high blood pressure, hyperthyroidism must be considered.

>> If the patient has high cholesterol and high blood pressure, the diagnosis of hypothyroidism should be considered.

Thyroid disease is common, and testing for it is simple, so everyone over age 35 should have a screening blood test. For more information on your thyroid, see *Thyroid For Dummies*, by Alan L. Rubin, MD (Wiley). Screening consists of a thyroid-stimulating hormone-level blood test.

TIP

Screening for thyroid disease begins at age 35 and is done every five years thereafter.

Hyperthyroidism and hypothyroidism can be treated easily:

>> **Hyperthyroidism:** You'll take medications by mouth to block thyroid hormone production or a dose of radioactive iodine.

>> **Hypothyroidism:** You'll take a replacement thyroid hormone by mouth. One pill a day keeps the person entirely normal — at least as far as the thyroid is concerned! That's as good a cure as I know.

In both conditions, the blood pressure returns to normal after treatment.

Sleep apnea

Sleep apnea is a condition in which an individual gasps for breath and snores during sleep following several stops in breathing. It's significant when it happens five or more times in an hour. The results of the restless sleep are extreme fatigue during the day, headaches, and a tendency to fall asleep when you don't want to, such as when driving a car and at work.

Because the lack of breathing occurs many times, you have a reduction in blood oxygen and an increase in carbon dioxide. The decrease in oxygen causes constriction of the blood vessels, resulting in high blood pressure. People with sleep apnea also tend to have an increased risk of heart disease.

Sleep apnea is diagnosed in a sleep laboratory where doctors can observe you sleeping, snoring, and failing to breathe for many periods of time. After the diagnosis, you use a continuous positive airway pressure (CPAP) machine when you sleep. The pressure provided by the CPAP machine (through a mask) keeps the airway open so you don't experience breathing loss, loud snoring, or gasping for air. Sleeping is much more restful, and you don't fall asleep during the day. The high blood pressure usually subsides as well. (Talk about a win-win situation!)

If the condition has gone on for a long time, your high blood pressure may continue, and pills may be required to control it.

2

Considering the Medical Consequences of High Blood Pressure

IN THIS PART . . .

Find out which organs are affected by uncontrolled high blood pressure.

Understand how high blood pressure affects the heart.

Get clear on the role of high blood pressure in kidney disease.

Think clearly about high blood pressure and the brain.

See the facts about high blood pressure and the eyes.

Chapter **5**

Protecting Your Heart from Heart Disease

Heart disease is the leading cause of death throughout the world. It involves the muscles of the heart and the blood vessels that provide nutrition to those muscles. Various forms of heart disease include *angina* (chest pain caused by a decreased blood supply to the heart) and *heart failure* (when your heart isn't able to pump enough blood or when the heart is unable to relax enough maintain an adequate flow to and from the body tissues). A *heart attack* occurs when there is death of heart muscle tissue due to a loss of blood supply). High blood pressure plays a critical role in the development of heart disease.

High blood pressure — especially combined with diabetes, smoking, and lack of exercise — can increase a person's chances of having a fatal heart attack by as much as 15 to 20 times. In fact, people with untreated high blood pressure may live 10 to 20 years less than people without high blood pressure. Bottom line: Your life span is lengthened when your blood pressure is controlled.

This chapter tells you what you need to know about high blood pressure and your heart. After reading this chapter, you'll understand how important blood pressure control is for your heart.

Taking your blood regularly, using the proper technique, is really important. Turn to Chapter 2 to find out how to measure your blood pressure.

Introducing the Mighty Heart: Pumping and Relaxing

The heart is a remarkable organ! It is mostly muscle and is about the size of a clenched fist weighing about 10½ ounces. This mighty muscle literally helps to "pump you up" — it's responsible for supplying blood and oxygen 24/7 to all parts of the body.

Your heart is located in your chest cavity behind your breastbone and between your lungs. It's divided into four chambers: the left and right atria (plural of *atrium*) and the left and right ventricles. Having a fundamental understanding of how the heart works is important if you want to understand how the heart can be affected by high blood pressure. Here's the play-by-play of how the four chambers of the heart work together:

>> The right atrium receives blood through a really large vein called the *vena cava* and pushes the blood into the right ventricle. The vena cava is the big vein that all the smaller veins flow into, kind of like the way small streams can flow into a larger river.

>> The right ventricle squeezes and sends the blood into the pulmonary arteries to the lungs, where the blood picks up oxygen. After the right ventricle squeezes the blood into the pulmonary artery, it takes a little time to relax and fill up with blood from the right atrium so it can squeeze again. It must be boring to be a ventricle!

>> After the blood picks up the oxygen as it travels through the lungs, the blood then goes to the pulmonary veins, which carry the blood back to the left atrium, which sends the blood down to the left ventricle.

>> The left ventricle squeezes the blood into the *aorta* (the major artery that sends the blood to every cell and organ in the body). Think of the aorta as the trunk of a tree with branches that flow into every organ of the body. The left ventricle also needs to time to relax and let the blood flow in so it can squeeze again.

How do your ventricles get the time they need to squeeze, relax, and fill? Via the valves that close, blocking backward flow, preventing the blood from going backward (from the left side of the heart to the lungs, from the right side of the heart to the veins, and from the ventricles to the atria).

The heart pumps approximately 1½ gallons of blood forward every minute. Each hour, it sends about 90 gallons around the body, enough to fill a car's 15-gallon gas tank six times. During a restful day, your heart pumps 2,160 gallons of blood. And when you're working or exercising, the number gets much higher.

The combination of the heart, the blood vessels that carry the blood, and the blood itself is called the *cardiovascular system*.

REMEMBER

Even though you have four chambers of the heart, the one chamber doctors pay really close attention to is the left ventricle because it pushes blood to the rest of the body. Over time, high blood pressure can cause changes to the integrity of the left ventricle, affecting its ability to squeeze and pump the blood, as well as relax and fill — the left ventricle can become unable to fully relax. This is a major way that high blood pressure affects the heart.

High blood pressure affects the heart in a few different ways:

>> It's a major risk factor for the development of coronary artery disease.

>> Over time, uncontrolled high blood pressure makes the heart work harder, resulting in a thickening of the heart muscle called *hypertrophy*. Hypertrophy is often described medically when talking about the left ventricle, often termed *left ventricle hypertrophy*.

Coronary artery disease and hypertrophy both increase the risk of development of congestive heart failure, which I discuss later in this chapter. High blood pressure, left ventricle hypertrophy, coronary artery disease, and congestive heart failure often occur together. Coronary artery disease and congestive heart failure are also the most common reasons adults are admitted (and readmitted) to the hospital.

Blocking Blood Flow to the Heart Muscle

Just like any other organ of the body, your heart muscle must receive oxygen, *glucose* (blood sugar), and other nutrients for optimal performance. These nutrients are the food and fuel for the heart muscle.

In *arteriosclerosis* (hardening of the arteries), deposits of cholesterol and formation of *plaque* (consisting of inflammatory cells and fibrous tissue) cause an affected artery to narrow and become partially obstructed, which affects the flow of blood to that artery. The heart muscle then becomes partially starved, which can cause pain. A complete obstruction causes a heart attack.

Figure 5-1 shows the location of the major arteries that provide blood supply to the heart muscles:

>> The right coronary artery supplies blood to the right side of the heart.

>> The left main coronary artery supplies blood to the left side of the heart. It, in turn, divides into the following:

- The left anterior descending artery, which supplies the front of the left side

- The left circumflex artery, which curves around to the back

>> Both the left and right coronary arteries arise as the left ventricle continues into the aorta.

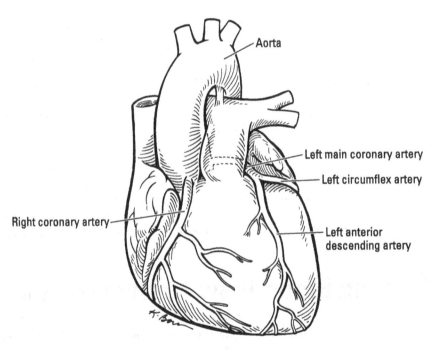

Illustration by Kathryn Born, MA

FIGURE 5-1:
Blood supply to the heart.

THE FORMATION OF PLAQUE

Arteriosclerosis begins with the formation of plaque. But how does this plaque form in the first place? When high blood pressure, smoking, diabetes, or increased levels of cholesterol (especially low-density lipoprotein [LDL] cholesterol) damage the inner lining of the arteries, a plaque begins to form. The following figure shows the parts of a normal artery before and after plaque develops.

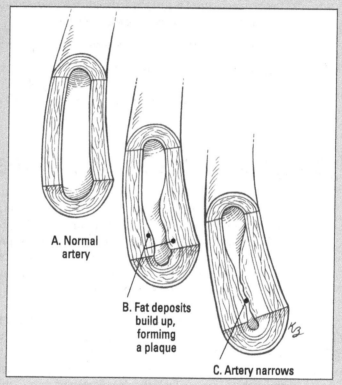

A. Normal artery

B. Fat deposits build up, formimg a plaque

C. Artery narrows

Illustration by Kathryn Born, MA

After damage occurs, the following steps take place:

1. Fat begins to accumulate within the *intima* (the innermost layer of the artery wall).

2. The chemicals that normally prevent changes to the fat can't reach it — the fat begins to change to a more damaging form.

(continued)

(continued)

3. White blood cells enter the intima, transform into *macrophages* (large cells), and begin gobbling up the changed fat, turning the cells into *foam cells*.

   Note: Macrophages normally remove waste products, harmful microorganisms, and foreign material from the bloodstream.

4. Calcium also deposits in the walls of plaque. It's responsible for the calcification in arteries that is visible in X-rays.

5. This accumulation of foam cells and calcium is now plaque. It grows and begins to stick out into the *lumen* (the hollow part) of the artery.

6. Blood flow to the heart muscle is reduced when 80 percent of the lumen is blocked.

7. Blood platelets can accumulate to form clots on the irregular surface of plaque. The clot can stay at that position (reducing the opening of the lumen even more) or break off and lodge in a smaller artery (completely closing off blood flow beyond it).

Analyzing Coronary Artery Disease

As atherosclerosis of the coronary arteries worsen and the arteries become more narrowed, a person can develop symptoms of chest pressure called *angina*. This significant symptom is typically described as a chest pressure feeling like an elephant is sitting on your chest. Other symptoms that are associated with coronary artery disease include nausea, sweating, jaw pain, tooth pain, and/or arm pain with or without chest pressure being present.

WARNING

Heart attack in women can have different symptoms than it does in men. Men often describe chest pressure that radiates to the arm or chest. Women often describe persistent nausea, fatigue, not "feeling right," sweating, or even weakness. If you're a woman and you're having any of these other symptoms, don't dismiss them, especially if they're persistent.

WARNING

Approximately one in five individuals can have a silent heart attack, without having any of these symptoms. This means that there is heart damage, but the patient isn't aware anything has happened.

REMEMBER

Coronary artery disease is a leading cause of increased mortality and morbidity in the United States and many countries around the world. According to the Centers for Disease Control and Prevention (CDC), one out of every five deaths in the United States every year is due to a fatal heart attack. In fact, in the United States about one person dies from heart disease approximately every 30 seconds. It's the leading cause of mortality among men, women, and most ethnic groups in the United States.

Understanding angina and heart attack

In this section, I cover coronary artery disease, which encompasses stable angina, unstable angina, and heart attack (technically called myocardial infarction).

Stable angina

Many individuals with coronary artery disease have angina, a relatively stable form of chest pain that doesn't worsen over time. Stable angina is chest pain that begins with activity and is relieved with rest. People most often feel the pain in the front of the chest on the left side and radiating down the left arm. It tends to be in the same area for an individual every time they have it. In some individuals, the chest discomfort can occur after a meal (when blood is diverted to the gastrointestinal tract) or during excitement. Strong emotions can also cause chest pressure, even without activity. For some people, symptomatic *discomfort* in the chest area is described as burning, squeezing, pressing, aching, or indigestion.

Other places where the pain occurs may include only the right side of the chest, or the left shoulder, and sometimes the right shoulder. It can also be felt in the jaw or even the tooth in some people. These non-classic presentations of chest pressure are referred to *anginal equivalents* and should not be ignored.

Some people may not manifest symptoms of chest pressure at all. This can occur in some individuals with diabetic neuropathy, which may prevent them from feeling the classic symptoms of chest pain.

The discomfort may last no longer than a few minutes, especially if you rest as soon as it starts. It doesn't last longer than 30 minutes.

Nitroglycerin taken under the tongue often reduces or stops the pain. In fact, this response helps to make the diagnosis — if nitroglycerin doesn't help the pain, it may be caused by something else.

Unstable angina

If stable angina is chest pressure or discomfort that occurs after exercise or activity and resolves with rest, then unstable angina is chest pressure or discomfort that occurs even at rest. The chest pressure may spontaneously go away on its own, or it may be relieved with nitroglycerin.

WARNING

Unstable angina that requires a more urgent evaluation by a health-care practitioner. If you're having episodes of recurrent or persistent unstable angina, get it evaluated as soon as possible — you may even need to go to an emergency room for more urgent evaluation and treatment.

Heart attack

In a heart attack, the plaque that has formed over time becomes unstable and causes a cascade of events, which cause the artery to become blocked. In a heart attack, heart muscle tissue dies because it lacks a supply of blood.

WARNING

A heart attack is an emergency and requires urgent hospital intervention. If you're experiencing symptoms of a heart attack, call 911.

Getting a diagnosis

If you're having episodes of stable or unstable angina, talk to your doctor. The doctor may use certain blood tests to characterize the type and extent of your heart disease, including the following:

>> **Cardiac enzymes (often referred to as troponin levels):** Blood chemicals that are in higher amounts when the heart damage is acute (when you're in a hospital setting or in the emergency room).

>> **C-reactive protein (CRP):** A substance in the blood that indicates a higher level of inflammation. CRP is often tested on an outpatient basis as part of a cardiac risk assessment (to determine your risk of having or developing coronary artery disease).

>> **LDL:** A form of fat in the blood that increases atherosclerosis. This test is often part of a lipid panel that a health-care provider would order in either an outpatient or inpatient setting. LDL is an important target of treatment because higher levels can promote atherosclerosis, which promotes coronary artery disease in the first place. Lowering your LDL level is important not only to prevent coronary artery disease from occurring in the first place but also to prevent it from getting worse.

For someone with stable angina and no sign of a heart attack, a health-care provider may recommend the following two tests, which evaluate the function and viability of your heart muscle under a controlled "stress" environment:

>> **Stress test:** During a stress test, you walk on a treadmill at increasing speeds and increasing slopes while a continuous *electrocardiogram* (ECG) — a recording of the electrical impulses in the heart) — is performed. There are characteristic changes on the ECG that may identify that a potential blockage or area of ischemia is present that normalizes when the activity is stopped.

>> **Myocardial perfusion scan (MPS):** The MPS is a specialized type of heart imaging study that evaluates the blood flow to the heart during stress to

better evaluate if a blockage or area of inadequate blood supply is present. This test shows where the heart muscle is and isn't receiving normal blood flow. After a special kind of tracer is injected through an IV, a device locates the tracer and is able to follow its path in the heart. When no radioactivity is observed, no blood delivery is occurring during that time.

TIP

There are other ways for a health-care provider, usually a cardiologist, to perform a stress test if you aren't able to walk on a treadmill or physically perform any strenuous activity. They can stimulate the heart activity enough to simulate physical activity and get a better look at your heart. Your health-care provider will discuss different testing options.

If stress testing/MPS indicates that there is a blockage(s) or areas of inadequate blood flow, more definitive testing may be ordered to better look at your heart anatomy and try to identify where the blockages may be. These tests include the following:

>> **Coronary angiogram:** This test is the gold standard for the diagnosis of coronary artery disease, and it's ordered when the previous tests indicate an abnormality. To find the areas of narrowing, the doctor places a catheter in the individual coronary arteries and injects a dye that's visible on an X-ray.

Coronary angiography may also be performed in the following situations:

- To further evaluate angina, especially if it isn't responding to medical treatment

- To help further define whether coronary artery disease is present, especially if the symptoms and/or prior testing aren't fully definitive

- If you have a history of coronary artery bypass surgery and symptoms are returning

- If you have an abnormal heart rhythm because of a blockage that needs to be further evaluated

If you go to the emergency room with persistent and significant chest discomfort and an ECG indicates that a coronary artery is significantly blocked, you'll be taken right to the cardiac catheterization lab for a coronary angiogram with the goal of doing angioplasty.

>> **Echocardiogram:** This is a specialized kind of ultrasound of the heart. A device that sends a sound wave to the heart muscle is held over your heart, producing a picture of the moving heart muscle (similar to the image pregnant women get of their babies). The echocardiogram is able to evaluate how well all four chambers of your heart are working at any given time (paying particular attention to the left ventricle). It's noninvasive and can be done in an outpatient or inpatient setting.

If a coronary angiogram clearly points to obstructive coronary artery disease, the doctor determines a treatment plan, taking into account how well the heart is functioning based on echocardiogram results.

Considering treatment options

Three major forms of treatment are available for coronary artery disease: medication and lifestyle modifications, angioplasty, and bypass surgery. Each has its advantages and disadvantages, and I cover them in the following sections.

Medication and lifestyle modifications

One treatment option for patients with stable, uncomplicated, nonobstructive coronary artery disease is medication and lifestyle modifications.

There are several classes of medications that a cardiologist (heart specialist) may prescribe in the treatment of coronary artery disease:

>> **Beta blockers:** Drugs that decrease the heart's oxygen requirements. Beta blockers slow down the heart and can increase your life span after a heart attack. Examples include propranolol, metoprolol, and atenolol.

>> **Calcium channel-blocking agents:** Drugs that decrease the heart's oxygen requirements by reducing blood pressure and heart rate. Examples include verapamil and diltiazem. Other medications in this class (including amlodipine) not only help to lower blood pressure but also prevent angina.

>> **Anticoagulants:** Drugs that prevent the blood's platelets from forming a clot. Examples include aspirin, clopidogrel, and ticagrelor.

>> **Long-acting nitrates:** Drugs that decrease the frequency of angina attacks by helping to dilate the blood vessels. They're available as pills as well as patches (the medication is absorbed through the skin). Examples include isosorbide dinitrate and isosorbide mononitrate.

>> **Nitroglycerin:** A drug that relieves symptoms of angina over a short period of time by dilating the blood vessels. It's taken under the tongue and usually works in minutes.

REMEMBER

Before prescribing drugs, your doctor will want to eliminate contributing factors (see "Recognizing and Treating Important Risk Factors," later in this chapter).

Angioplasty

Angioplasty — technically called percutaneous coronary artery angioplasty (PTCA) — is often recommended for a single blood blocked vessel.

During angioplasty, you're awake but given enough sedation to help you remain calm and relaxed during the procedure. There are two options for accessing the blocked artery: through the femoral artery (in the groin) or through the radial artery (in the wrist). Your cardiologist will make a tiny incision to find the artery and insert a guide wire and a tube up to the area of blockage. They'll observe the blocked artery by injecting dye through the tube and taking an X-ray. Then they'll inflate a balloon at that end of the tube to widen the area of the blockage and stretch it out. This step may be repeated, and then the tube and balloon will be removed.

After the blockage is opened, the cardiologist may also place a *stent* (an open tubular structure) to act like a scaffold and keep the artery open. The stent is coated with a medicine to help prevent platelets from collecting there. You may be in the hospital for one day after the procedure to monitor your status; you're typically able to return to work the following week.

Angioplasty can't be performed if an artery is completely blocked. It also isn't effective when many separate blockages are present.

Bypass surgery

If multiple vessels are affected by coronary artery disease, bypass surgery — technically called coronary artery bypass grafting (CABG) — is often recommended.

During a bypass, you're placed under general anesthesia and a large incision is made to open the chest. The flow of blood is diverted from the heart to a heart-lung machine, which provides blood to the rest of the body while the heart is still. The surgeon attaches a healthy blood vessel (often a vein from the leg or the inside of the chest) onto both sides of the blocked artery. The blood then flows freely through that blood vessel. The surgery can take several hours, especially if several arteries are being repaired. After the procedure, you're monitored in the intensive care unit (ICU) for a few days; an average hospital stay for this type of surgery is approximately one week.

Bypass surgery is not without risk of complications (including heart attack, stroke, infection, and even death), especially in patients over 70 years old and those with other conditions such as chronic kidney disease and diabetes.

Developing Congestive Heart Failure

Uncontrolled high blood pressure is a significant contributing factor in the development of congestive heart failure. If high blood pressure is allowed to continue, the heart — especially the left ventricle — gets bigger and thicker over time. It can only thicken so much before it's unable to fill and/or relax effectively, which leads to the development of heart failure.

In the following sections, I cover the signs and symptoms of congestive heart failure and then get more into the nitty-gritty of the main causes of this condition.

Noticing important signs and symptoms

The most common symptom of congestive heart failure is shortness of breath. Often, breathing is only initially difficult during exercise or any type of physical activity. As heart failure worsens, however, you may have difficulty breathing while at rest.

When your doctor asks you about shortness of breath, they'll try to getter a better sense of how bad it is. You may be asked how long it takes before you develop shortness of breath when walking at a brisk walking pace. If you have stairs in your house, you may be asked how many stairs you're able to go up before you develop shortness of breath and how this is different from a few months ago.

TIP

You may also be asked if you've altered your activities (for example, maybe you now sleep downstairs because you get too short of breath going up the stairs). In the days leading up to your appointment, make a list of ways you've changed your routine to compensate for shortness of breath.

Sometimes the heart failure is significant enough that you may be unable to lie down without raising the head of your bed or using multiple pillows. Lying flat causes a condition called *orthopnea*, which is worsening shortness of breath that improves when you sit up or raise your head.

Sometimes a severe coughing spell and shortness of breath that can't be relieved just by sitting up or raising the head may wake you up. This condition, called *paroxysmal nocturnal dyspnea*, can be a terrifying experience because you can't catch your breath. It's caused by an abundance of fluid in the lungs, which is associated with congestive heart failure.

WARNING

Symptoms as severe as paroxysmal nocturnal dyspnea require a call to 911 and emergency room treatment.

If you experience shortness of breath, confusion, severe fatigue, or the new onset of chest pain, call your health-care provider. If you're unable to catch your breath and the chest pain does not go away, call 911.

Understanding what your doctor will look for

Here are some of the signs and symptoms that a health-care provider will look for if they suspect you may have congestive heart failure:

>> **Swollen legs:** The legs swell because of *edema* (water in the tissues). You can sometimes see a dent when the finger pushes into the skin on the front of the legs. This is a significant sign of fluid retention in the setting of heart failure.

>> **Enlarged liver:** If the heart is unable to pump the fluid forward, it can back up into the liver and cause an enlarged liver, which can sometimes be painful. The medical term for this condition is *congestive hepatopathy*.

>> **Extra heartbeats:** In congestive heart failure, the heart has to deal with extra fluid, so your doctor will listen with their stethoscope for an extra heartbeat due to the extra fluid the heart has to deal with.

>> **Rales:** This is a crackling type of sound in the lungs that your doctor can hear with a stethoscope. It indicates the presence of fluid in the lung tissue, which is a sign of congestive heart failure.

>> **Abdominal swelling:** Some people retain fluid in their legs, but others may note a more swollen belly area. They may note their pants are tighter or they're using fewer belt holes than before.

>> **Decreased urine:** If you have congestive heart failure, you may be urinating less than before. If the heart failure is severe, it can affect blood flow to other organs of the body, including the kidneys, which can decrease the amount of urine you make on a given day.

Determining the underlying cause of heart failure

Under the influence of high blood pressure, the heart muscle begins to thicken just like any muscle that constantly does more work. About 20 percent of people with high blood pressure have *left ventricular hypertrophy*, a severe version of this condition, which can lead to heart attacks and/or heart failure. As the muscle gets thicker, it loses its elasticity, which affects the ability of the heart to pump and relax. The more uncontrolled the high blood pressure, the worse these symptoms become.

Decreasing pump function

REMEMBER

The main job of the left ventricle is to pump the blood to the aorta and to the rest of the body. When the heart is unable to squeeze and pump the blood to the rest of the body, it can cause many of the symptoms covered earlier.

The ability of your heart to work as a pump can be assessed with a specialized ultrasound of the heart called the echocardiogram. It is used to calculate how well your heart is able to pump the blood with each heartbeat called the *ejection fraction* (or EF for short). A normal EF is about 65 percent (meaning that if the heart ultrasound says that the EF is 65 percent, this means that your heart is pumping at 100 percent capacity).

TIP

If you have received care from a health care provider, you have access to your medical records and are able to see notes about your medical condition(s) from your health care provider(s). You are being introduced to different medical terms in this chapter and throughout this book as these are important and very common medical terms that you may see and sometimes knowing a little bit of the common technical jargon used can be incredibly helpful.

Being unable to chill out and relax

For many years the primary focus of congestive heart failure was on the pump function of the heart. While this is important, believe it or not it is not the most common reason for congestive heart failure. It is actually a failure of the heart to relax. Recall from earlier in the chapter that the heart has to relax in order to be able to fill with blood first to be able to then pump it to the rest of the body. In order the relax the walls of the ventricle have to be able to relax and expand a little bit to allow the heart to fill.

One of the consequences of uncontrolled high blood pressure and hypertrophy of this left ventricle is that the thickened heart muscle is unable to fully relax. The heart muscle is thickened and it becomes stiff like a board; the inability of the heart to fully relax is the most common cause of heart failure called diastolic heart failure. Common causes of this condition, as you may be able to guess include uncontrolled high blood pressure for many years and/or coronary artery disease.

TIP

You are going to be introduced to a couple of more technical terms here just to pull this altogether. Systolic heart failure is the decreased ability of the heart to function effectively as a pump; this means that the ejection fraction of the heart is reduced as measured by a cardiac focused ultrasound or echocardiogram (see "Getting a diagnosis," earlier in this chapter, for more on echocardiograms).

REMEMBER

Congestive heart failure can arise from a variety of problems (not just high blood pressure), including issues with the valves of the heart (mitral valve, for example), endocrine conditions, and other systemic conditions that can affect the heart.

Treating congestive heart failure

If you're diagnosed with congestive heart failure, your cardiologist will prescribe medications and lifestyle modifications (see the next section). Some important recommendations may include the following:

>> **Significant reduction in your intake of sodium and sugar:** This helps not just to lower blood pressure but to prevent water retention associated with increased salt.

>> **Medications:** Some of the medications your doctor may prescribe include the following

- A drug from the category of *ACE inhibitors* (see Chapter 13) to help lower blood pressure and help improve heart function and to help reduce sodium and water retention early in the development of heart failure

- Diuretics to help eliminate excess fluid

- Beta blockers to help improve heart function

- A special medication called valsartan-neprilysin

- Blood pressure control

>> **Physical activity and exercise:** You'll likely perform these activities under the guidance of your health-care provider. Your activity may be initially restricted until things are more stable.

>> **Weight loss:** This helps to reduce how hard your heart has to work.

>> **Restriction of fluid intake:** You may be told to drink no more than 48 ounces of fluid daily.

Recognizing and Treating Important Risk Factors

Although medications are important for the management of high blood pressure, coronary artery disease, and congestive heart failure, a more important aspect is lifestyle modification. This section focuses on four fundamental risk factors intrinsic to these conditions.

REMEMBER

Uncontrolled high blood pressure makes both heart failure and heart attacks much more difficult to manage, so controlling the high blood pressure is an early step toward managing these complications.

Some risk factors that contribute to high blood pressure can't be avoided (like a family history of early heart disease). But doing everything possible to avoid or eliminate other risk factors helps to prevent heart failure and heart attacks — two complications of high blood pressure — and minimize their impact if they do occur.

Reducing high cholesterol

High cholesterol levels are an important risk factor for the development of heart disease and often go hand in hand with high blood pressure. This condition is very treatable and commonly involves the use of dietary modifications (see Chapter 9). If you have documented heart disease, your doctor will also talk to you about medications such as statin therapy to help keep your cholesterol levels low.

REMEMBER

Your doctor will order a test called a fasting lipid panel. Although there are several components to this panel, the initial focus is on LDL cholesterol. If you have heart disease, the goal is to get this number below 70.

Quitting smoking

In many ways, smoking is a greater problem than high cholesterol. It increases inflammatory risk of coronary artery disease by several times. This is such an important topic that Chapter 11 discusses this topic is greater detail.

REMEMBER

In terms of benefits to your health, nothing you do is of greater value than quitting smoking.

Controlling diabetes

Coronary artery disease is the most frequent cause of death among those with diabetes. The extent of cardiovascular disease and of the *atherosclerotic plaque* (areas of obstruction in blood vessels) in those with diabetes results in a poor response to angioplasty and the need for bypass surgery when angina or a heart attack occurs.

Diabetes is diagnosed when the blood glucose level is 126 milligrams per deciliter (mg/dL) on two or more occasions in the fasting state or 200 mg/dL in a random blood glucose check on two or more occasions. However, you have *impaired fasting glucose* (commonly known as prediabetes) if your fasting blood glucose is 100 mg/dL to 126 mg/dL in the fasting state or 140 mg/dL to 200 mg/dL at random. The increased risk of heart disease associated with blood glucose is present in people with prediabetes as well.

REMEMBER

Prediabetes can be reversed and diabetes can be prevented. If your blood glucose puts you in the prediabetes range, talk with your doctor about steps you can take now to prevent diabetes.

TIP

If you have diabetes, keep your fasting blood glucose as close to the normal range as possible (between 80 mg/dL and 125 mg/dL) and keep your *hemoglobin A1c* (which tests glucose control over a three-month time frame) less than 7 percent if possible.

REMEMBER

Keep your weight down, get plenty of exercise, avoid fats, and keep your blood glucose under 126 mg/dL fasting or 140 mg/dL after eating a meal. These steps keep your heart risk at a minimum. See the excellent book *Diabetes For Dummies*, 2nd Edition (Wiley), for full details on controlling diabetes.

Stepping up physical activity

Lack of physical activity is a risk factor for heart disease. If you work in a job where you're sitting most of the day, get up and walk around at least once each hour. This small intervention can add to your lifespan. Other options include using a standing desk. The key is purposeful movement every hour.

REMEMBER

Don't forget to include your regular daily exercise, such as walking and/or strength training. Turn to Chapter 12 for more information.

IN THIS CHAPTER

» Cleaning house: Your kidneys' filtering systems

» Understanding how kidneys affect high blood pressure

» Discovering how high blood pressure impairs renal function

» Recognizing common causes of chronic kidney disease

» Treating end-stage renal disease

Chapter **6**

Caring for Your Kidneys

The kidneys play an important role as the body's great filter. In this chapter, I explain how high blood pressure affects the kidneys, as well as how the kidneys affect blood pressure. I start by introducing the basic functions of the kidneys, the important hormones that the kidneys produce, and common conditions that can affect kidney function. I also review some critical aspects of chronic kidney disease.

The kidneys are, indeed, wonderful organs. After reading this chapter, you'll likely have the same great appreciation for your kidneys that I have for mine. You may even raise a glass of water and toast them!

REMEMBER

Don't accept a diagnosis of high blood pressure until you've had at least three blood pressure readings obtained, and even then, measure your blood pressure at home with a reliable monitor (see Chapter 2) both to confirm the diagnosis and to follow your body's response to treatment. Be sure to take your blood pressure the correct way because technique definitely affects your blood pressure reading. The importance of taking your blood pressure on a regular basis can't be emphasized enough, especially if you've been told you have kidney disease.

Examining the Role of Your Kidneys

Your body has two kidneys, each weighing about 6 ounces (or less than 0.5 percent of the body's total weight). Each kidney is approximately 4 inches high, 2 inches wide, and 1 inch thick. Figure 6-1 shows the kidneys' position in your abdomen. They're found in the back part of your belly, on each side of your spinal column, right under your ribs, where the middle of your back meets your lower back.

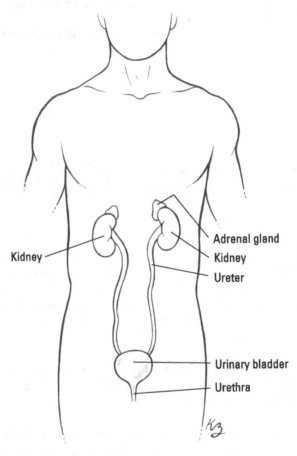

FIGURE 6-1:
The position of the kidneys.

Illustration by Kathryn Born, MA

Each kidney connects to a long tube called the *ureter*. The kidneys make urine, which flows through the ureter into the *bladder* (a container that stores the urine temporarily). When the bladder is full, it empties into the *urethra*, and that's your cue that you need to empty your bladder. The kidneys, ureters, bladder, and urethra form the *genitourinary tract* (GU tract).

The kidneys are made up of many parts. Blood enters the kidneys through the large *renal arteries.* The *renal cortex* is the kidney's outer shell, which contains blood vessels and urine tubes. The *renal pyramids* (the innermost tissue of the kidneys) contain the urine tubes and the specialized tissue that permits fine-tuning of the various substances that leave the kidneys in the urine. Figure 6-2 shows an inside view of some of the kidney's major parts.

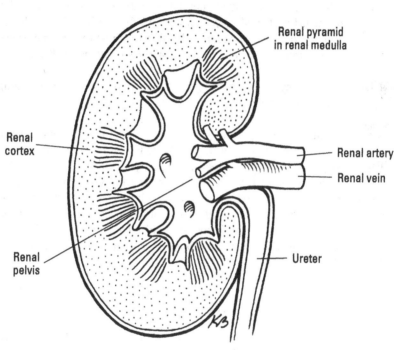

FIGURE 6-2:
The internal parts of the kidney.

Illustration by Kathryn Born, MA

In the following sections, I explain the filtering function of the kidneys, as well as review the important hormones the kidneys make and how they're related to blood pressure.

Filtering

Your kidneys are truly amazing. Your digestive tract only eliminates the waste that goes through the digestive tract, but the kidneys do so much more. They filter the blood, which acts much like a cargo ship as it picks up waste from all the cells in your body. The blood carries the waste to your body's "filtration headquarters" — the kidneys.

Your kidneys filter an enormous amount of blood every minute, about 1½ quarts. Picture a water filter that you may have on your kitchen sink. The water flows into the filter where toxins (normal waste products) are removed. In the same way, the blood flows through specialized filters in the kidneys that remove the toxins. In the body, the product of the filtered material is urine, which you eliminate every time you make a pit stop in the bathroom (well, almost every time). The kidneys reabsorb the important minerals (like sodium, potassium, and magnesium) and other important body elements back into the body instead of letting them escape in the urine. The kidneys can keep all these minerals in balance — not too much and not too little. The kidneys' ability to adjust the levels of these minerals in your body is important in promoting balance and good health.

Your kidneys aren't just big filters; each kidney is actually composed of a million small filters called *nephrons*.

Sodium is an important *electrolyte* (a mineral that has a natural electric charge). The amount of sodium in your body is regulated by your kidneys. If you've been diagnosed with high blood pressure, your health-care provider has likely talked with you about the importance of limiting your sodium intake. This is because restricting your sodium intake is an important aspect of treating blood pressure. Most doctors recommend a limit of 2,000 mg of sodium per day. One important way to know how much sodium you're consuming on a daily basis is to read food labels for their sodium content. For more on sodium restriction, turn to Chapter 10.

Making hormones

In addition to being the body's great filters, the kidneys have other important functions as well. Your kidneys make a few important hormones that are important in regulating blood pressure, preventing anemia, and maintaining optimal bone health. Here's a list of some of the key hormones produced by the kidneys:

>> **Renin:** As I mention earlier, the kidneys have "sensors" that can determine the levels of different minerals and electrolytes in the body. An important one is sodium; when the kidneys sense that the sodium content in the blood is low or if the blood pressure is low, they need a fail-safe mechanism in which to help your body conserve the sodium it needs. These signals send a sensor to a specialized part of the kidney to produce a hormone called *renin*. Renin does two important things:

- It helps to raise the blood pressure.

- It stimulates the adrenal glands to produce a hormone called *aldosterone,* which asks your kidneys to conserve and hold onto the sodium and water that it needs.

When the sensors of the kidney perceive that the blood pressure has improved, they stop making renin.

Renin and aldosterone are blood tests that your health-care provider may order to evaluate resistant high blood pressure (see Chapter 4). These are the main two "blood pressure hormones" that you read a lot about in this book because they're so important.

>> **Erythropoietin:** Specialized cells within the kidneys produce *erythropoietin,* a hormone that stimulates the bone marrow to make more red blood cells. Whenever blood is lost or a trip to high altitude demands more oxygen, the need for red blood cells is greater, so the kidneys produce erythropoietin. When kidney function declines, anemia develops because the kidneys are less able to make this important blood-producing hormone.

>> **1 alpha hydroxylase D:** This enzyme converts vitamin D to its more active form in the kidney. When kidney function declines, the kidney is less able to convert vitamin D to its most active form, 1,25 hydroxyvitamin D3. The amount of highly active vitamin D3 decreases. As a result, calcium isn't taken up in sufficient quantities, and bone health is affected. 1,25 dihydroxy vitamin D can be prescribed to help maintain bone health.

REMEMBER

Not only is vitamin D important for bone health, but it also has effects on other body systems as well. For example, it helps with making your immune system work better and it can help in the management of anemia.

The connection between vitamin D and high blood pressure is an area of ongoing investigation. Scientists think vitamin D helps the blood vessels work better and may help in the management of high blood pressure. Many people are deficient in vitamin D3; your vitamin D3 level can be measured by a simple blood test. If you haven't had your level measured, talk with your health-care provider.

Understanding Chronic Kidney Disease and Common Causes

Chronic kidney disease affects one in every seven individuals, or approximately 40 million people in the United States. It's no surprise that high blood pressure is a leading cause of kidney disease, but the opposite is also true: Kidney disease is the leading cause of resistant high blood pressure (see Chapter 4). The following sections explain how your kidneys and blood pressure affect each other.

Defining chronic kidney disease

If the main role of your kidneys is to work as your body's filter, kidney disease is any condition that compromises your kidneys' ability to effectively act as a filter.

Chronic kidney disease has many potential causes, but two of the most common are diabetes and high blood pressure. But no matter the cause of kidney disease, managing blood pressure is important to preventing it from getting worse.

WARNING

How does high blood pressure affect kidney function? Over months to years, uncontrolled high blood pressure causes progressive damage and scarring to the kidneys.

REMEMBER

You can have chronic kidney disease *not* caused by high blood pressure, but high blood pressure can still be a problem. This is because when you have chronic kidney disease, your kidneys have fewer filters, and those filters need to work harder for your kidney to be able to do its job. High blood pressure causes more damage to the kidneys and can worsen kidney function.

People can have stable chronic kidney disease for years without any change in their kidney function. It depends on the cause of the kidney disease, but many other factors, including control of high blood pressure are important in preventing kidney disease from worsening.

Diagnosing chronic kidney disease

Your health-care provider can tell if your kidney function is compromised by doing some blood tests — specifically, testing your creatinine level and your blood urea nitrogen (BUN) level. They'll also order some basic urine tests — urinalysis and testing the urine for albumin (the most abundant protein in the body). Identifying the presence of protein in the urine is important no matter the cause of chronic kidney disease, because if *proteinuria* (protein in the urine) is present, it's a significant risk factor for worsening kidney disease.

WARNING

With proteinuria, the kidney must work harder to break down the protein and filter it. This causes scarring and damage to the kidneys, in a similar way to how uncontrolled high blood pressure affects the kidneys, but even more so. That's why catching proteinuria early is important.

A *nephrologist* (kidney specialist) may need to do some other testing, including a kidney ultrasound (to see the size and shape of the kidneys), specialized blood and urine tests, and sometimes even a kidney biopsy to determine the exact cause of what's affecting the kidneys.

WARNING

Many people aren't even aware that they have chronic kidney disease — the initial sign that someone has it is often abnormal bloodwork. In fact, some signs and symptoms of kidney disease may not show themselves until the kidney function is less than 15 percent!

TIP

That said, there are some signs you should pay attention to that can signal that you may have a kidney problem that may be present even in earlier stages of chronic kidney disease:

>> The presence of "bubbly" or "frothy" urine can signal that your urine is leaking protein it isn't supposed to.

>> Blood in the urine (called *hematuria*) can be present and may signal a problem in the kidney or anywhere along the entire genitourinary tract. If you see tea-colored urine, call your health-care provider for further evaluation.

>> Swelling in the legs, also referred to as *edema,* can be a consequence of proteinuria seen in advanced chronic kidney disease (where the kidney function is so poor such that the kidneys have difficulty getting rid of extra salt and water, which can cause swelling).

TIP

If your health-care provider has diagnosed you with chronic kidney disease, ask to review your lab tests with them. Keep copies of your lab tests so you can keep track of your kidney health as well.

Staging and treating chronic kidney disease

If you've been told that you have chronic kidney disease, the next most common question is, "How bad is my kidney function?" There are five stages of chronic kidney disease, with each stage representing a further decline in kidney function. Stages I and II represent mild kidney disease, stage III is moderate, and stages IV and V are advanced.

Table 6-1 outlined the stages of chronic kidney disease and the treatment options.

TABLE 6-1	Stage of Chronic Kidney Disease and Treatment Options	
Stage	Kidney Function	Treatment Options
I	90% or more (but proteinuria is present)	Control blood pressure if it's abnormal. Use medication to lower proteinuria (see Chapter 13). Possibly see a nephrologist for further evaluation of proteinuria.
II	60%–89%	Control blood pressure if it's abnormal. Use medication to lower proteinuria (see Chapter 13). Evaluate potential causes of chronic kidney disease. Possibly see a nephrologist for further evaluation of proteinuria.
III	30%–59%	Consult a nephrologist for further evaluation and management of kidney disease.
IV	15%–29%	Continue working with a nephrologist. Discuss dialysis and transplant options.
V	Less than 15%	See "Coping with End-Stage Renal Disease" later in this chapter.

Coping with End-Stage Renal Disease

End-stage renal disease occurs at Stage V (see the preceding section), when you have less than 15 percent of kidney function. The kidneys can't perform their primary function as an effective filter, so toxins build up and excess fluid is retained.

Currently, more than 700,000 people in the United States are being treated for end-stage renal disease, with approximately 500,000 on dialysis. High blood pressure and diabetes account for approximately 65 percent of those on dialysis.

REMEMBER

The course of chronic kidney disease is different for everyone. If you reach a stage V, you won't necessarily need to start dialysis. At this stage, you're closely followed by a nephrologist. The decision to start dialysis is based on the presence of certain symptoms, including the following:

>> Fatigue and weakness

>> Easy bruising

>> Constant itching

>> A metallic taste in the mouth

>> Breath that smells of urine

- » Shortness of breath (even while sitting still, but even more with minimal activity)
- » Nausea and vomiting
- » Weight loss
- » Decreased appetite
- » Increased leg swelling
- » Decreased urine output
- » Cramping and spasms in the legs (especially at night while trying to sleep)
- » Irritability and/or confusion
- » Hiccups

You can have any or many of these symptoms. They normally subside after treatment with dialysis begins.

WARNING

If you have kidney disease and you take medications, the dosage of some of your medications may need to be adjusted if you start dialysis.

Dialysis

Dialysis is an artificial filter that does the job that the kidneys are no longer able to perform. Nephrologists think of dialysis as a temporary bridge for the person to eventually get a kidney transplant (if they're eligible for one).

REMEMBER

The key point you should take away from this section is that you have options regarding dialysis. The main ones include *peritoneal dialysis* or *hemodialysis*. I cover both of these in the following sections.

REMEMBER

The decision regarding the type of dialysis you'll do is not just an educated decision based on preference but also a personal one. Everyone is wired differently and knows what they can and can't do. These are delicate conversations that take time — that's why a discussion about dialysis options usually begins when a person enters stage IV of chronic kidney disease.

Peritoneal dialysis

If you have end-stage renal disease, one option is peritoneal dialysis, which takes advantage of the filtering capacity of your abdominal cavity (called the *peritoneum*). The peritoneum prevents the passage of larger elements of the blood, such as blood cells and protein, but allows the liquid part, with all its dissolved substances, to pass through.

Peritoneal dialysis is an important option discussed by nephrologists and is very much advocated by the nephrology community for the following reasons:

>> It can be done at home. The patient is in charge of their own treatments, including control of their schedule. Dialysis revolves around the patient's daily life — their daily life doesn't have to revolve around dialysis.

>> Because it's done every day (often several times a day), it's very well tolerated with minimal side effects.

>> The patient is able to live their life and travel (with the caveat that planning is needed ahead of time so they have the necessary supplies for their trip).

>> The dietary restrictions are minimal and often can be more liberal compared to hemodialysis.

Peritoneal dialysis consists of the following steps:

1. **A surgeon places a permanent catheter into the abdominal cavity.**

2. **A *dialysate* (salt-and-sugar solution) is inserted into the abdominal cavity through the catheter.**

3. **Because of their high concentration, body wastes enter the dialysate solution.**

4. **The dialysate, along with the unwanted wastes, is drained out through the catheter.**

Each cycle of putting in and removing dialysate is an *exchange*. Figure 6-3 shows a peritoneal dialysis.

There are two types of peritoneal dialysis:

>> **Continuous ambulatory peritoneal dialysis** uses gravity to fill and empty the abdomen. Usually the individual needs three to four daytime exchanges and maybe one during sleep.

>> **Continuous cycler-assisted peritoneal dialysis** uses a machine to fill and remove the dialysate from the abdomen, especially during the night to make the overnight dialysis more efficient. Three to five exchanges take place during sleep. Another, longer exchange may take place during the day using a higher concentration of sugar to promote more waste removal.

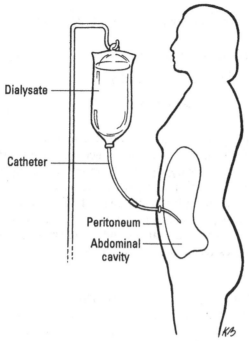

Dialysate

Catheter

Peritoneum

Abdominal
cavity

FIGURE 6-3:
The technique of
peritoneal
dialysis.

Illustration by Kathryn Born, MA

**TECHNICAL
STUFF**

The success of peritoneal dialysis depends on:

>> How much dialysate can be placed into the abdominal cavity

>> How rapidly the wastes pass into the dialysate

Testing the dialysate, as well as the patient's blood and urine, once a month determines the efficiency of each exchange. Measurement of the waste products in these three fluids determines whether the patient needs more dialysis, more solution, a different amount of sugar in the solution, or all three adjustments.

Some people can't do peritoneal dialysis because their peritoneum doesn't allow sufficient rapid passage of body fluids. In this case, hemodialysis may be the preferred method of treatment. Other reasons why some people can't do peritoneal dialysis include:

>> The presence of inflammatory bowel disease or other acute gastrointestinal conditions

>> Inability to do self-care or lack of a caregiver

>> Extensive prior abdominal surgery with many scars

Here are some other reasons why you may *choose* not to pursue peritoneal dialysis:

>> You may not want to be trained on the techniques of peritoneal dialysis.

>> You may not want to do dialysis every day.

>> You may not have room for the dialysis supplies.

WARNING

Proper training in peritoneal dialysis technique is essential because, when it's done incorrectly, you're at increased risk of developing *peritonitis* (an infection of the fluid in the abdominal cavity). Peritonitis raises body temperature. The abdomen may be tender and swollen and you may be nauseated and vomit. The fluid that's drained from the abdominal cavity, the dialysate, becomes cloudy instead of clear, and bacteria may grow out from it. If you notice these symptoms, call your doctor right away. Peritonitis is treatable and usually responds well to antibiotics. However, it sometimes recurs, and the bacteria infect the catheter. Then a new catheter is needed.

TIP

When you're on dialysis, you're never alone. There is a peritoneal dialysis dedicated nurse on call 24 hours a day if you need advice or help, and there is always a nephrologist or advanced practitioner specialized in nephrology on call to help you when needed.

Hemodialysis

During hemodialysis, your blood circulates through a specialized filter called a *dialyzer*. There are two different options for hemodialysis:

>> **In-center hemodialysis:** Dialysis is done at a dedicated outpatient dialysis center, usually three times a week for three to four hours at a time.

>> **Home hemodialysis:** Short hemodialysis treatments are done four to five days a week at home. This type of dialysis is slower and easier than what's done at outpatient dialysis centers.

The most important part in the preparation for hemodialysis is the creation of specialized vascular access often in the nondominant arm. Ideally, a surgeon performs a minor operation in which an artery and a vein are connected to form an arteriovenous *fistula* (a connection between the two). The fistula heals in approximately two to three months and then is ready to be used when dialysis is needed. The planning and creation of a fistula takes time — this is why these discussions occur when you're in stage IV.

Many times, dialysis needs to be started earlier and sometimes even more urgently. In those situations, a more urgent access is required, and a surgeon or radiologist would place a catheter that would be used for hemodialysis, with the ultimate goal being the creation of a fistula.

The process of hemodialysis occurs in the following manner:

1. **Needles are placed in the artery of the fistula (to deliver blood to the machine) and the vein of the fistula (to return blood to the body).**

2. **The blood from the artery enters the dialyzer and passes through filters called the dialyzer.**

3. **Wastes are removed while normal body components are retained or returned to the blood.**

4. **The blood returns to the body through the needle into the vein.**

Figure 6-4 shows the technique of hemodialysis.

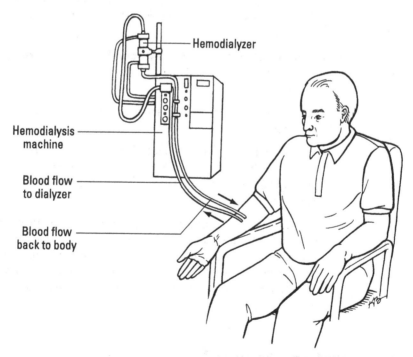

FIGURE 6-4:
The technique of hemodialysis.

Illustration by Kathryn Born, MA

Just as in peritoneal dialysis, the fluid produced by hemodialysis and the patient's blood can be tested to evaluate the adequacy of the treatment.

Hemodialysis, like peritoneal dialysis, has its share of advantages and disadvantages. Advantages include the following:

>> **It can be done at home, at a dialysis center, or within the hospital.** Treatment at home allows you to set your own schedule as long as you follow your doctor's recommendations. Treatment at a hospital ensures that professional help is available in case it's needed. Also, because patients usually receive dialysis as a group, they often enjoy being in the company of other patients with similar problems.

>> **It takes considerably less time than peritoneal dialysis.**

Disadvantages of hemodialysis include the following:

>> **You must follow a fairly careful diet.** You have to avoid fluids (depending on how much urine you're making), salt, foods that contain phosphorus (like milk, cheese, and chocolate), and foods that contain potassium (like citrus and tomatoes).

>> **Having the treatment done away from the home requires planning.** You often have to contact a dedicated outpatient dialysis center and see if there is an open space available.

>> **With home dialysis, the dialysis machine and equipment take up space in the home.**

>> **With home dialysis, you and another person must be trained to administer and monitor it.** For example, you need to know how to clamp off the needles if bleeding occurs and you must be vigilant about caring for the fistula to prevent infection.

>> **Hemodialysis in an outpatient dialysis center occurs three days a week for 12 hours total.** This is contrast to the kidneys working 24/7. It can be difficult for many people to tolerate because the treatment time is shortened to only approximately 12 hours totals. Some individuals may not tolerate hemodialysis at all and skip treatments; others may be exhausted on dialysis treatment days.

Kidney transplant

When possible, transplantation is the best answer to end-stage renal disease. You end up with a new, healthy kidney that performs like your *good* old kidneys.

In kidney transplantation, you receive a new kidney from a living donor or from a donor who has recently passed away. The preparation and testing for a kidney transplant take time; the testing is extensive. If you're getting a kidney from a donor who has recently passed away, your name goes on a waiting list.

As shown in Figure 6-5, during a transplant, the kidney is placed in your lower abdomen during a surgery that takes several hours. The failed kidneys are usually left in the body unless they're infected, extremely large, and taking up space (in the case of an inherited condition such as polycystic kidney disease) or causing high blood pressure. Arteries in the new kidney are attached to your own arteries. As Figure 6-5 shows, the ureter is transplanted to your bladder as well. The new kidney may make urine instantly, or it may take hours, days, and even sometimes weeks to make urine. Hospitalization post-surgery lasts a few a days or longer based on recovery of kidney function, as well as the time it may take to recover post-operatively.

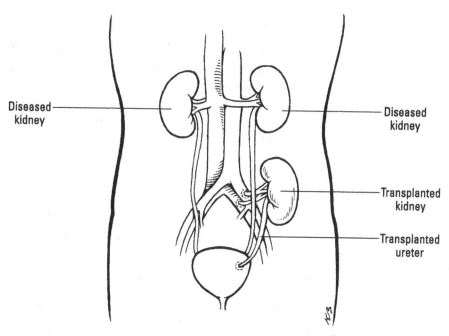

Diseased kidney

Diseased kidney

Transplanted kidney

Transplanted ureter

FIGURE 6-5:
The appearance of a transplanted kidney in your abdomen.

Illustration by Kathryn Born, MA

Ninety percent of transplanted kidneys (whether from family members or unknown donors) still function after one year and 80 percent function after five years. On average, kidneys from living donors survive 15 years, and kidneys from donors who have died last an average of about 10 years.

Before you're eligible for a transplant, you must

>> Be well enough to withstand surgery and take medications to prevent rejection.

>> Be willing and able to take the medication without fail.

>> Not have other conditions that prevent successful transplantation (such as cancer in the last two years, severe heart disease, or severe lung disease).

>> Have a good support structure to help you.

Due to health reasons, only half of the patients on dialysis are eligible for a kidney transplant.

Kidney transplantation is a long-term solution with these significant advantages:

>> Patients feel as normal as they did before they became sick.

>> No dialysis is necessary as long as the kidney continues to function.

>> Patients only need to follow a few dietary restrictions if the kidney function of the transplanted kidney is not normal.

Like all treatments, however, things to be aware of regarding kidney transplantation include the following:

>> Transplantation requires major surgery.

>> Few kidneys are available, so if you have to wait for a donor, it may be a long wait, sometimes years. In the meantime, dialysis is necessary.

>> Some transplants fail, so a second transplant is needed.

>> Patients need to take medications called *immunosuppressants* for the rest of their lives to prevent their bodies from rejecting the transplanted kidney. These drugs have side effects such as the promotion of diabetes and the weakening of the immune system (making infection more likely).

>> The drugs or rejection of the new kidney may be responsible for high blood pressure (present in up to 90 percent of transplant survivors), which can further damage the new kidney.

TIP

If you're on the list for a transplant, be ready to go at a moment's notice. Have your bag packed and transportation available, and be prepared to stay in the area of the transplant center for up to four weeks. Check out the transplant center before you go by checking the database of the Scientific Registry of Transplant Recipients at https://srtr.transplant.hrsa.gov/. Find out:

>> The center's experience

>> The survival of the center's transplants

>> Other services (support groups and assistance with travel and housing)

You'll be amazed by how many centers are available. For instance, California and Texas have 26 centers each that do kidney transplantation, and New York has 14. You'll find a wide range of experiences among those centers.

Chapter **7**

Keeping Your Brain Intact

U ncontrolled high blood pressure can affect the brain in a couple of different ways, but one of the most common ways the brain is affected is from a stroke. According to the World Stroke Organization, globally, stroke is the second major cause of disability and death together. Significant risk factors for stroke include high blood pressure, *hyperlipidemia* (high cholesterol and triglycerides), smoking, diabetes, and obesity. According to the Centers for Disease Control and Prevention (CDC), one out every three adults in the United States has at least one of these modifiable risk factors.

Stroke doesn't just affect the elderly. In fact, according to the CDC, in 2014, more than one-third of individuals admitted to the hospital for a stroke were under 65 years of age.

A stroke occurs when blood flow to a part of the brain is blocked. There are two different types of strokes: ischemic and hemorrhagic. An ischemic stroke occurs when there is a blockage of blood flow in a blood vessel; a hemorrhagic stroke occurs when there is bleeding in the brain. Depending on the severity of the stroke, affected individuals may experience significant neurological symptoms, including *focal weakness* (weakness affecting one side of the body or weakness in a particular extremity — either an arm or a leg) and/or impaired vision and speech, numbness, and/or tingling in their face and/or extremities. A severe stroke can also cause permanent paralysis.

REMEMBER

Think of a stroke as a "brain attack." As with a heart attack, time is of the essence in terms of getting treatment as soon as possible after symptoms develop.

In this chapter, I explore the different causes of a stroke, as well as its presenting signs and treatment. I also explain other ways that high blood pressure can affect the brain. Although stroke treatment is important, stroke prevention is even more important. For even more information, check out *Stroke For Dummies,* by John R. Marler (Wiley).

TIP

Each of the organs that high blood pressure can affect are discussed separately in this part, but high blood pressure can affect all these important organs simultaneously. The danger of uncontrolled high blood pressure is that you may not have any symptoms until a sudden event occurs, such as a stroke. Be proactive with your health, especially your blood pressure.

TECHNICAL STUFF

Unless otherwise specified, in this chapter I use the term *stroke* to refer to acute stroke.

Understanding the Causes of Strokes

Up until the 20th century, it was believed that a stroke was as random an event as being struck by lightning. The word *apoplexy* derives from a Greek word meaning "to be thunderstruck," and many people used the term *apoplexy* to refer to what we know as a stroke today. Because a stroke was considered to be unpreventable, it was also referred to as a *cerebrovascular accident.* But we know that most, if not all, strokes aren't "accidents" — you can do a lot to reduce your risk of having a stroke.

In this section, I fill you in on the different causes of strokes.

Atherosclerosis

Atherosclerosis (hardening of the arteries caused by a buildup of cholesterol deposits) can affect the heart (see Chapter 5), it can also affect the arteries leading into and within the brain. The most common cause of a stroke is due to blockage of blood flow to a certain part of the brain. If the blood flow ceases entirely, a stroke may occur. This type of stroke is called an *acute thrombotic stroke.*

The blood supply to the brain has multiple sources. (Figure 7-1 shows the unique circulation of blood in the brain.) The left and right cerebral arteries entering the skull in the front of the brain combine with the left and right vertebral arteries entering the skull in the back of the brain to produce a circle of blood supply called the *circle of Willis* at the base of the brain. Other arteries that make up the circle are also shown in Figure 7-1. If one of the arteries is blocked, blood from the other arteries can fill the circle and provide blood to all areas of the brain. In an ischemic stroke, viable brain tissue can die if circulation isn't opened within about four and a half hours.

REMEMBER

Ischemia refers to any cause that blocks blood flow to any vessel (heart, brain, kidney, and so on). In the brain, ischemic strokes account for approximately 90 percent of all strokes and the remaining 10 percent are due to hemorrhagic strokes. The two major types of ischemic strokes include *thrombotic* stroke (due to atherosclerosis) and *embolic* stroke (due to a blood clot).

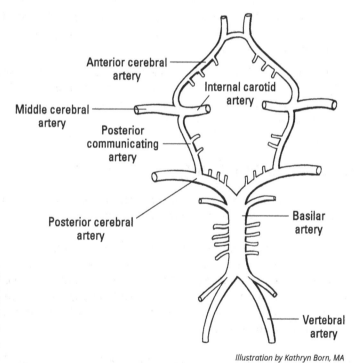

FIGURE 7-1:
The unique joining of separate blood vessels form the circle of Willis.

Illustration by Kathryn Born, MA

Cerebral embolus

Approximately 15 percent of all ischemic strokes are due to a cerebral embolus. A *cerebral embolus* is a *blood clot* (a solid mass of blood cells, protein, and other blood substances) or solid tissue that breaks off from an *atherosclerotic plaque* (an irregularity inside the artery due to the formation of a cholesterol deposit) that travels through the bloodstream into the brain. The bloodstream carries the atherosclerotic plaque particle from its site of origin — either from the heart or from other sites, including the large arteries in the neck — into the arteries of the brain, where it becomes wedged and blocks circulation to part of the brain.

One of the most common causes of a cerebral embolus is due to an abnormal heart rhythm called *atrial fibrillation* (uncoordinated twitching movements of the heart), with the embolus commonly arising from the left atrium of the heart. Here's how this may happen:

1. The heart is normally in what is called *sinus rhythm* (the normal lub-dub sound of the heart like a one-two beat) that loses its regular beating pattern and gives way to atrial fibrillation.

2. The left atrium is not contracting (no lub, just the dub). The heart's left atrium fails to completely empty its blood into the left ventricle. The blood that remains is able to form clots and can break off and travel the bloodstream into the arteries of the brain.

If someone is admitted to the hospital for a stroke, part of the evaluation often includes getting a specialized ultrasound of the heart called an echocardiogram (see Chapter 5) to evaluate the heart to see if there is a clot in the atrium, as well to evaluate the heart function.

Brain hemorrhage

Brain hemorrhage (bleeding within the brain or between the skull and the brain) accounts for approximately 10 percent of strokes.

Two-thirds of brain hemorrhages occur within the brain. As a result of high blood pressure or other disease conditions, the muscular wall of the artery may weaken and form one or more *aneurysms.* An aneurysm looks like a balloon attached to the artery, and like a balloon, it can burst and subsequently bleed into the brain. Because the brain doesn't have space to make room for the extra blood, brain tissue is squeezed and may die.

The other one-third of brain hemorrhages actually occur *outside* the brain in a space called the *subarachnoid space* (the thin separation between the inside of the bony skull and the outside of the brain's fleshy gray matter). Bleeding within this space usually results from an aneurysm that forms inside the skull but outside the brain. If the aneurysm ruptures, the blood flows around the brain, causing increased pressure and a severe headache that's often described as the "worst headache of my life."

HYPERTENSIVE EMERGENCY WITH ENCEPHALOPATHY: IT'S NOT A STROKE

Hypertensive emergency is an acute medical condition in which the blood pressure is very elevated (with the systolic blood pressure [the top number] more than 180 mmHg and/or the diastolic blood pressure [the bottom number] more than 100 mmHg). In the brain, this elevated blood pressure can cause an acute hemorrhagic stroke (see "Brain hemorrhage," in this chapter) or a type of confusion called *encephalopathy* that is treated by lowering the blood pressure.

Because the presentation of acute hypertensive encephalopathy in a hospital setting can mimic an acute stroke — confusion or altered mental status can be seen in both — brain imaging is essential in differentiating between the two. To rule out stroke, a health-care practitioner will order either a CT scan of the brain or an MRI of the brain to make sure no acute bleeding is occurring.

Other causes of bleeding in the brain can include trauma (such as hitting your head after a fall). The risk of bleeding dramatically increases if you're on a blood thinner (such as aspirin, clopidogrel, ticagrelor, or coumadin) and/or direct oral anticoagulants (such as rivaroxaban or apixaban).

Another cause of brain hemorrhage can be very highly uncontrolled blood pressure. This can be an acute small bleeding stroke in the areas of the brain stem, as well as other brain structures including the pons and the thalamus. This kind of bleed is often seen on brain imaging studies (discussed later in this chapter).

Preventing Stroke

High blood pressure is the most important risk factor in the development of a stroke, and controlling blood pressure can prevent stroke. High blood pressure contributes to the development of a stroke in several ways, including promoting and accelerating the development of atherosclerosis. Many clinical trials have demonstrated that lowering blood pressure can reduce the incidence of strokes.

But high blood pressure is just one risk factor for stroke. In this section, I cover other important risk factors and let you know what you can do to further reduce your stroke risk.

Understanding the risk factors you can't change

Some risk factors for stroke you can't do anything about:

>> **Age:** The older you are, the higher your stroke risk.

>> **Sex:** At any age, strokes tend to occur more often among men than women, but women are more likely to die when they have strokes than men are.

>> **Family history:** If one or more of your parents or siblings has a history of a stroke, you're at increased risk.

>> **History of prior stroke:** If you've had a stroke before, you're at increased risk of having another one.

Modifying the risk factors you can

Reducing the risk factors you can control can make a huge difference in reducing your stroke risk. These risk factors include the following:

>> **Alcohol consumption:** Reducing alcohol consumption decreases stroke risk (see Chapter 11).

>> **Atherosclerosis:** Lifestyle modifications and certain medications can help reduce your risk of developing atherosclerosis (see Part 3).

>> **Atrial fibrillation:** If you have atrial fibrillation, it can be brought under control with the help of the right treatment (see the nearby sidebar).

>> **Diabetes:** The high blood glucose levels of uncontrolled diabetes associated with high blood pressure and high cholesterol can be brought under control. Check out *Diabetes For Dummies*, 6th Edition, by Simon Poole, Amy Riolo, and Alan L. Rubin (Wiley), for more information.

>> **Excess weight and obesity:** Even if you're only ten pounds overweight, that excess ten pounds contributes to high blood pressure. However, dieting and exercising can reduce your weight.

>> **High blood cholesterol:** Cholesterol increases the risk of stroke. Diet, exercise, and medications, if necessary, can control this risk factor.

>> **Illegal drugs:** Using illegal substances such as amphetamines and cocaine increases blood pressure and your chances of developing a stroke.

>> **Lack of exercise:** A sedentary lifestyle predisposes you to a stroke, but exercise can drastically reduce your risk. Purposeful movement every day is important, especially if your job involves sitting most of the day.

ASSESSING AND TREATING ATRIAL FIBRILLATION

Atrial fibrillation is a significant risk factor for an embolic stroke. It's one of the most common *arrhythmias* (abnormal heart rhythms) that health providers see. How would you know if you had atrial fibrillation? Some individuals may notice ther heart racing at times (also known as *palpitations*). They may experience dizziness or lightheadedness that comes and goes. And they may take their pulse and notice a really fast heart rate. Other people may not have any symptoms at all.

When someone is being admitted to the hospital for a suspected or a confirmed stroke, because atrial fibrillation is a significant cause of stroke, obtaining a specialized ultrasound of the heart called an echocardiogram is automatically part of the diagnostic workup. If atrial fibrillation is discovered, treatment involves consultation with a cardiologist, who will prescribe medications to slow down the heart rate initially and talk with you about medications to thin the blood to lower stroke risk.

>> **Tobacco:** Smoking damages the walls of your blood vessels and accelerates atherosclerosis. Stopping this habit can help improve and restore your blood vessel health over time.

If you keep these risk factors under control, you're sure to decrease the likelihood of a disabling stroke.

Reducing stroke risk with medications

TIP

If you're at high risk to have a stroke, a number of drugs can lower the risk. The most commonly prescribed medications include the following:

>> **Aspirin:** Aspirin prevents platelets in the blood from forming a clot. If you have a transient ischemic attack (TIA) — often referred to as a "mini-stroke" — aspirin may reduce your risk of having a stroke by 30 percent. Talk with your health-care provider before starting aspirin.

>> **Clopidogrel (Plavix) or ticagrelor (Brilinta):** These antiplatelet drugs don't cause the gastrointestinal bleeding of aspirin, but their ability to reduce the risk of stroke is similar to aspirin's.

>> **Coumadin (Warfarin):** This anticoagulant prevents the formation of clots, but it comes with the risk of excessive bleeding. Anticoagulants must be monitored with blood tests. They're often given to reduce embolic risk if someone has atrial fibrillation.

Thinking F.A.S.T. When Suspecting a Stroke

The symptoms of an impending stroke can occur suddenly. Don't waste a minute getting to a hospital! You may prevent much of the damage if you receive treatment within the first four and a half hours.

REMEMBER

Memorize the F.A.S.T. acronym when it comes to recognizing the symptoms of a stroke. If you experience any of the following symptoms or see another individual displaying any of them, call 911:

>> **F:** Facial weakness, including facial drop on one side of the face.

>> **A:** Arm weakness on one or both sides of the body.

>> **S:** Slurred speech or difficulty speaking.

>> **T:** Time is tissue — the sooner a blocked artery can be opened up and blood flow can be restored, the better the outcome.

Other symptoms can include the following:

>> Sudden blurred or decreased vision in one or both eyes

>> Numbness, weakness, or paralysis of the face, arm, or leg on one or both sides of the body

>> Difficulty understanding or development of confusion

>> Sudden dizziness, loss of balance, or an unexplained fall

>> Nausea, vomiting, or and/or difficulty swallowing

>> Sudden headache and/or change in the pattern of headaches

DIFFERENTIATING TIA FROM STROKE

The symptoms of stroke may not last very long. Often, the symptoms resolve on their own without any interventions. When symptoms resolve on their own without any residual effects, the patient is thought to have experienced a transient ischemic attack (TIA).

In fact, the old definition of TIA was a neurologic deficit that lasted less than 24 hours and resolved on its own. When this definition was initially created, the brain imaging we used wasn't as sophisticated as it is today. The main way that health-care providers can differentiate a TIA from a stroke is through imaging findings like a brain MRI.

Utilizing Brain Imaging

Each area of the brain performs a certain function (see Figure 7-2). When a stroke occurs, the health-care provider (often in the emergency room) needs to be able to identify the damaged part of the brain to (a) localize the probable blocked or bleeding artery and (b) determine whether treatment is feasible.

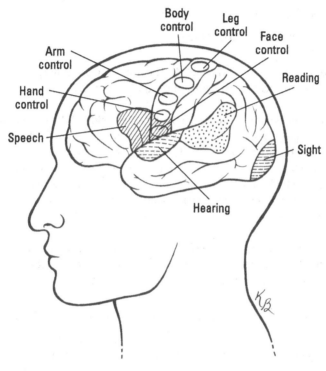

Illustration by Kathryn Born, MA

FIGURE 7-2:
Sites in the brain that control body functions.

Loss of blood supply to specific areas of the brain can result in the loss of a specific function and consequent signs and symptoms. Because the right side of the brain controls the left side of the body, and because the nerves cross over, careful *mapping* of the loss of function (noting the nerves that correspond) can determine the area of the brain that's damaged. For example, paralysis of the left leg means that the right brain leg control area is affected.

Some functions, like memory, however, are controlled by only one side of the brain. If the stroke affects the right side of the brain, for example, the victim may experience some of the following symptoms, in addition to weakness or paralysis on the left side of his body:

>> Tendency to be impulsive or disorganized

>> Lack of coordination and tendency to fall

>> Inability to remember

>> Lack of insight and judgment

If the stroke occurs on the left side of your brain, you may experience some difficulty communicating in addition to right-sided weakness or paralysis.

Other symptoms that aren't particular to one side of the body may follow a stroke. For example, the survivor may not see or think as they did before; their perceptions may be altered. As a result, they may be depressed or suffer mood swings — suddenly bursting into laughter for no apparent reason. In another instance, one side of the body may be weaker and vision on that side may be poorer. The individual may lose awareness of that side of their body and tend to bump into objects with that side.

REMEMBER

Your doctor may need to perform various sophisticated tests to clarify where the damage has occurred and why. The following list describes a few of the tests a doctor will commonly do in the emergency room:

>> **Computed tomography (CT)** is done to initially rule out a brain hemorrhage.

>> **CT angiogram** is a specialized study looking at the blood vessels of the head and neck to look for an obstruction, aneurysm, or narrowing that could account for the patient's symptoms and possibly be amenable to acute intervention.

>> **Magnetic resonance imaging (MRI)** can pinpoint the location of a stroke in the first 24 hours, examine minute areas of the brain, and differentiate between a TIA and a stroke. In addition, an MRI can look for aneurysms and malformations that can eventually cause a hemorrhage in the arteries and veins.

WARNING

You generally won't be able to have an MRI if you have any significant metal in your body — including a metallic implant or a pacemaker (although some pacemakers are MRI friendly).

>> **Doppler ultrasound tests** evaluate blood flow in an artery. Sound waves are directed to the artery (usually in the neck, looking at the carotid arteries [the arteries outside the brain]) to indicate whether blood is flowing slowly or normally.

Understanding Treatment Options for Stroke

When a stroke occurs, the *ischemic core* (area of restricted blood supply) suffers a permanent loss of brain cells. The *ischemic penumbra* (the larger area around that core) is still alive and can be saved with quick action using a *tissue plasminogen activator* (tPA; brand name: Activase) or another clot-dissolving drug to break up any clot or obstruction to the flow of blood. This drug must be used within the first four and a half hours after the stroke to really benefit the brain and prevent more tissue loss.

tPAs can't be used in a hemorrhagic stroke (see "Brain hemorrhage," earlier in this chapter) because it doesn't involve blood clots. Unfortunately, hemorrhage is an occasional side effect of tPAs, and patients who have received tPAs are closely monitored in the intensive care unit (ICU) of a hospital.

TIP

Patients who have had a stroke use anti-platelet medications such as aspirin and clopidrogel in order to prevent future stroke (see "Reducing stroke risk with medications," earlier in this chapter). They're usually on an aspirin for the rest of their lives.

In addition to medications, if someone comes to the hospital with a stroke, the following procedures may be followed:

>> An interventional radiologist who specializes in the neurologic system can sometimes perform a *thrombectomy* (removal of a thrombus) or *embolectomy* (removal of an embolus) and restore blood flow to the affected area.

>> If an aneurysm has ruptured causing bleeding in the brain, neurosurgery can stop the bleeding by clipping or tying off a bleeding aneurysm that's the source of the stroke. That may stop the bleeding and prevent it from rupturing. The decision to perform this procedure depends on the location of the aneurysm. It may not be possible without damaging important brain tissue.

>> A surgeon may perform an *endarterectomy* (a specialized surgery to remove a blockage often in the carotid arteries). During this surgery, the doctor opens the neck where the artery is blocked and removes the blockage. This surgery is done if there is evidence of significant blockage in the carotid arteries. *Note:* Even if surgery successfully repairs one blood vessel, it may not cure the problem because the brain's blood supply comes from so many blood vessels; others may also be obstructed.

>> Stents can be used in carotid artery blockage just as they are in coronary artery blockage (see Chapter 5). So far, though, studies haven't determined whether carotid endarterectomy or stenting is the better procedure.

Recovering from a Stroke

If you've had a stroke and symptoms that have persisted after the stroke, recovery is very important. The following sections provide some insights into the rehabilitation and recovery process after a stroke.

Regaining function

It can take some time after a stroke to determine how much function someone will be able to regain. The rehab process can begin within 24 hours of a stroke if you're stable enough. If you're unable to move your extremities on your own, passive range of motion exercises can be performed with the goal to maintain and restore mobility, flexibility, and strength to the affected extremity. You'll be encouraged to move as much as possible, and you'll work with physical and occupational therapists to initiate a program to try to regain as much functioning, mobility, and strength as possible.

Working with rehabilitation specialists

There are different options for rehabilitation for a stroke. Where you'll go after being discharged from the hospital will depend on many factors, including the severity of the stroke as well as your ability to be able to be safely discharged to a home setting with home-based therapies. The amount of family support available is also important (if you live alone and still requires assistance for activities of daily living, you may have to go to a rehab facility).

There are several options for rehabilitation:

>> **Therapy at home:** A physical and occupational therapist may come to your home if you're stable enough to live at home and going back and forth to the hospital would be difficult. The therapist can inspect your home environment and offer suggestions to improve your safety at home, decrease fall risk, and improve efficiency when it comes to activities of daily living.

>> **Inpatient rehabilitation unit:** Another opportunity for rehabilitation is in an inpatient rehabilitation unit. This option is great if you aren't yet able to go home and require a more intense level of rehabilitation. One requirement for the inpatient rehab unit is that you be able to participate in a more intense level of rehabilitation for three to six hours a day. Dedicated rehabilitation unit staff carefully analyzes your level of function and sets clear goals for restoration. You work with physical therapists, doctors, and specialized nurses to help regain your independence.

>> **Skilled nursing facility:** If you aren't yet able to go home but you don't qualify for an inpatient rehab unity, a skilled nursing facility is another option. They perform and provide rehabilitative and restorative services on a daily basis, as well as taking care of other medical needs.

>> **Outpatient rehabilitation unit:** If you can return home, you may be able to go to an outpatient unit for rehabilitation services. You'll visit the outpatient center to work with a team of specialists who design a personalized program for you.

IN THIS CHAPTER

» **Looking at the basic anatomy of the eye**

» **Understanding the effects of high blood pressure on the eye**

Chapter **8**

Eyeing Your Blood Pressure

N ot only are the eyes the window to the soul, but they're also the one organ of the body that can quickly provide clues to the evidence of other systemic conditions. Your health-care provider can look into your eye with a special "eye scope" called an *ophthalmoscope* and immediately get a glimpse of not only your eye health but also your overall health. Examples of conditions that show up in the eyes include diabetes and high blood pressure; in fact, the eye is the one organ that can show evidence of high blood pressure without doing any specialized imaging or lab testing.

TIP

One way your health-care provider can tell if you've had high blood pressure for a long time is by looking at your eyes as part of your physical exam. An annual physical exam is a great way for your health-care provider to keep an eye (no pun intended!) on you and your overall health.

In this chapter, you find all the information you need to better understand how high blood pressure affects the eyes, both in the short term and over the long term. But first, in order to understand how high blood pressure affects the eyes, you need a basic primer on the anatomy of the eye.

Eyeballing the Anatomy of the Eye

Figure 8-1 gives you a bird's-eye view of the basic anatomy of the eye.

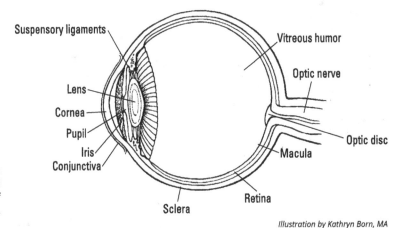

FIGURE 8-1: The internal structures of the eye.

As you can see, there is a lot going in there. The two aspects of this figure to focus on when it comes to high blood pressure are the retina and the optic disc:

» **Retina:** The retina represents the innermost layer of the eye. It contains certain types of eye receptors that are responsible for the detection of light and color. When light contacts these receptors, nerve impulses are generated. These nerve impulses are sent to specialized cells that form the optic nerve.

» **Optic disc:** The optic disc represents where nerves from the retina fuse with the optic nerve. Blood vessels that supply the retina first enter the optic disc.

In addition to receptors and nerve fibers, your retina also contains blood vessels. Like the blood vessels in the rest of your body, they deliver oxygen and necessary nutrients to your eyes.

Getting Hyper about Hypertensive Retinopathy

Your health-care provider or *ophthalmologist* (eye specialist) can use an ophthalmoscope to look at the blood vessels in the retina to see if there is evidence of *hypertensive retinopathy* (damage to the blood vessels in the eye caused by high blood pressure).

The process of arteriosclerosis that can occur in other blood vessels of your body (see Chapter 5) can affect your eye as well. This causes a thickening of the blood vessels in the eye, which, over time, affects your retina. Eventually, it can cause blurry or double vision and headaches.

One main difference between an eye exam done by your primary-care provider and an ophthalmologist is that the ophthalmologist will use special eye drops to dilate your eyes so they can see everything inside the eye. Ophthalmologists also have special machines to examine and test your eyes for many different conditions.

REMEMBER

While your eyes are dilated, they're very sensitive to light. You can't drive for a period of time after your eyes have been dilated, so you'll need to wear sunglasses and get a ride home.

Hypertensive retinopathy progresses through a series of four stages:

>> **Grade I:** In the first stage, your health-care provider will see narrowing of the retinal blood vessels.

>> **Grade II:** In the second stage, the narrowing of the retinal blood vessels is even more significant, such that the blood vessel in the eye can look as if it's being pinched or nicked.

>> **Grade III:** In the third stage, your health-care provider can see other changes in the retina and in the blood vessels, including swelling of the retina and the formation of very small *aneurysms* (dilated areas of the blood vessel) and/or small areas of bleeding in the retinal blood vessels.

>> **Grade IV:** In the fourth stage, a health-care provider can see swelling of the optic disc called *papilledema* (increased pressure in the eye, as well as increased pressure in the brain). Papilledema can be caused by other conditions besides uncontrolled high blood pressure, but high blood pressure

is the most common cause. Papilledema can be a chronic condition (due to longstanding worsening hypertensive retinopathy) or an acute condition (when there is a sudden increase in blood pressure; see Chapter 2).

WARNING

If your blood pressure is elevated and you're experiencing double vision or blurry vision, call 911. Do not drive yourself to the hospital.

Risk factors for the development of hypertensive retinopathy include age, the length of time someone has high blood pressure, and the severity of the high blood pressure. Other risk factors include tobacco use and family history of high blood pressure.

Another risk factor is diabetes, which can dramatically affect the eyes and also cause a condition called *diabetic retinopathy* (changes that occur in the vessels of the eyes over time due to high blood glucose levels). In many cases, diabetes and high blood pressure overlap and the same organs that are affected by high blood pressure are affected by diabetes, including the eyes.

REMEMBER

If you have hypertensive retinopathy, this is even more reason to do all that you can do to control your blood pressure.

3

Preventing and Treating High Blood Pressure

Find foods that lower high blood pressure.

Kick salt and sugar to the curb.

Quit smoking and reduce your intake of alcohol and caffeine.

Get moving to lower your blood pressure.

Look at the plethora of high blood pressure medications and find one that works for you.

See what new research is showing us about high blood pressure.

IN THIS CHAPTER

» Getting the lowdown on the DASH diet

» Meditating on the Mediterranean diet

» Pondering the importance of plant-based nutrition

» Shaving off a few pounds with diet

» Getting support from a nutritionist

Chapter **9**

Choosing Foods That Lower High Blood Pressure

You've heard the adage that you are what you eat. Well, when it comes to managing high blood pressure, that's one old saw to keep in mind. Focusing on diet is important when you're trying to lower your blood pressure. Plus, when you make the most of the foods your body takes in, you'll lose weight naturally (if you need to) because you're providing your body with the nutritional benefits it needs.

In this chapter, I fill you in on several nutritional approaches to healthy eating. From the DASH diet to the Mediterranean diet to the plant-based approach, these nutrition plans do more than just help to lower your blood pressure; they also reduce inflammation, improve the health of all your organs, and having organ-protective benefits as well. Healthy eating — combined with lowering your sodium and sugar intake (see Chapter 10) — can really help to lower your blood pressure. Plus, you'll feel better at the same time!

DASHing Down Your Blood Pressure

Even after more than two decades, the well-reviewed DASH diet is still a mainstay nutrition plan for the treatment of high blood pressure. Based on initial study results at four major medical centers in the United States, the Dietary Approach to Stop Hypertension (DASH) diet was published in the *New England Journal of Medicine* in 1997. All individuals on the DASH diet successfully reduced their systolic and diastolic blood pressure (see Chapter 2 for more about these terms).

Table 9-1 shows the average reduction in millimeters of mercury for the systolic blood pressure and the diastolic blood pressure for participants who followed the DASH diet.

TABLE 9-1   ## Average Reduction in Systolic and Diastolic Blood Pressure on the DASH Diet

Group	Systolic Blood Pressure (mm Hg)	Diastolic Blood Pressure (mm Hg)
African Americans	6.9	3.7
Caucasians	3.3	2.4
Established high blood pressure	11.6	5.3
No high blood pressure	3.5	2.2

Are you intrigued? In the following sections, you read about how the DASH diet was created and how you can get started on the DASH diet.

Leading up to DASH

DASH was created when doctors noted that vegetarians generally have lower blood pressure and a lower incidence of coronary artery disease (see Chapter 5) and stroke (see Chapter 7) than nonvegetarians do. The big difference between vegetarians and nonvegetarians is that vegetarians eat more fruits and vegetables than nonvegetarians do. They also, of course, eat no meat and generally have less cholesterol and saturated fat in their diet.

Because a vegetarian program isn't a practical recommendation for everyone, scientists tried to replicate the vegetarian program while permitting some meat. They looked for the substances in the foods vegetarians eat that could explain the fall in blood pressure.

The scientists recognized that a nutritional program with more fruits and vegetables has more potassium, which definitely affects blood pressure. The higher the potassium, the lower the blood pressure. So, the increased potassium may be a partial explanation for vegetarians' lower blood pressure, but it's not the *entire* story because similar amounts of potassium don't lower the blood pressure to the same extent unless the intake of sodium is also reduced.

The other important nutrients in vegetables and fruits are calcium and magnesium. Early studies regarding magnesium consumption and high blood pressure were conflicting, but magnesium supplementation does help dilate the blood vessels and helps to maintain the health of the blood vessels. Magnesium supplementation is also necessary if you're on diuretics used to treat high blood pressure (see Chapter 13), because these medications can cause your body to lose magnesium and potassium.

WARNING

If you have chronic kidney disease or other medical conditions (like diabetes) that may predispose you to high potassium levels, talk with your health-care provider about which fruits and vegetables are lower in potassium and which are higher. Talk with a nutritionist to help design a nutrition plan that's right for you.

The creators of the DASH nutrition plan felt that the mix of different nutrients is likely responsible for their blood-pressure-lowering effect. They performed a study to evaluate the effects of the DASH diet on blood pressure.

Proving the value of DASH

The study involved 459 people with a systolic blood pressure under 160 mm Hg and a diastolic blood pressure of 80 to 95 mm Hg. In addition, the study participants:

>> Were all older than 22

>> Had no history of taking medications for high blood pressure

>> Had to stop taking all vitamins and food supplements

>> Had to limit their alcohol consumption

>> Couldn't have poorly controlled diabetes, high cholesterol levels, or have a body mass index (BMI) greater than 35

For three weeks, the participants closely followed a common standard American diet (high in fats and total calories). They were then randomly assigned into three treatment groups:

>> The first group continued consuming the standard American diet.

>> The second group consumed a diet higher in in fruits and vegetables.

>> The third group followed the DASH diet.

After only two weeks, the group consuming the standard America diet showed no change in blood pressure, while the group consuming fruits and vegetables lowered their blood pressure. The group consuming the DASH diet, however, had the *greatest* reduction in blood pressure, and they maintained this reduction for the entire study.

The average reduction in the DASH group's blood pressure was 6 mm Hg systolic and 3 mm Hg diastolic, but the best results were among the people with the highest blood pressure — 11 mm Hg systolic and 6 mm Hg diastolic. Other studies using DASH have demonstrated other benefits, including lowering total cholesterol and low-density lipoprotein (LDL) cholesterol (the "bad" kind).

DASH-Sodium, a second study that used various levels of sodium with the DASH program, showed that the lowest sodium level consumed (1,500 mg per day) lowered blood pressure even more.

Getting with the program

The DASH program is traditionally based on a 2,000-calorie-per-day diet. In the following sections, I provide you with the foods and servings in the program, sample menus, and tips for getting started and sticking with it.

Specific foods and servings

REMEMBER

The 2,000-calorie DASH eating plan consists of the foods and servings shown in Table 9-2. If you need to consume fewer calories, use the lower number of servings; if you need more calories, use the higher number of servings.

TABLE 9-2   **DASH Eating Plan Servings**

Food Group	Number of Servings	Serving Size Examples	Good Food Choices
Grains and grain products	7–8 per day	1 slice of bread; ½ bagel; ½ cup dry cereal; ½ cup cooked rice, pasta, or other cereal	English muffins, high-fiber cereals, oatmeal, pita bread, and whole-wheat breads
Vegetables	4–5 per day	1 cup raw, leafy vegetables; ½ cup cooked vegetables; 6 ounces vegetable juice	Artichokes, broccoli, carrots, collards, green beans, kale, peas, potatoes, spinach, squash, sweet potatoes, tomatoes, and turnip greens
Fruits	4–5 per day	6 ounces fruit juice; 1 medium fruit; ½ cup dried fruit; ½ cup fresh, frozen, or canned fruit	Apples, apricots, bananas, dates, grapefruit, grapefruit juice, grapes, mangos, melons, orange juice, oranges, peaches, pineapples, prunes, raisins, strawberries, and tangerines
Dairy products (low-fat or nonfat)	2–3 per day	1 cup 1% milk; 1 cup low-fat yogurt; 1½ ounces nonfat cheese	Buttermilk (skim or low-fat), cheese (nonfat and part-skim mozzarella), milk (skim or 1%), yogurt (nonfat or low-fat)
Meat, poultry, or fish	2 or fewer per day	3 ounces cooked lean meat, fish, or poultry	Lean meats, poultry without skin, and nothing fried or sautéed
Fats	2½ per day	1 teaspoon oil, butter, margarine, or mayonnaise; 1 tablespoon regular salad dressing; 2 tablespoons light salad dressing	Olives, olive oil, avocadoes, dark chocolate, nuts, and seeds
Nuts, seeds, or legumes	4–5 per week	⅓ cup nuts; 2 tablespoons seeds; ½ cup cooked legumes; 3 ounces tofu	Almonds, garbanzo beans, kidney beans, lentils, mixed nuts, navy beans, peanut butter, peanuts, pinto beans, sesame seeds, split peas, sunflower seeds, tofu, and walnuts
Sweets	5 per week	1 tablespoon sugar; 1 table-spoon jelly or jam; ½ ounce jelly beans; 8 ounces lemonade	Fruit smoothies, yogurt, apple crisps, any frozen fruit, applesauce, dark chocolate

Sample menus

To make up your daily nutrition, Table 9-3 shows a sample menu.

Consider filling your own menu out following Table 9-4, or plan an entirely different day of meals, as Table 9-5 shows.

TABLE 9-3   A 2,000-Calorie DASH Menu

Breakfast	Lunch	Dinner	Snack
3 grains	1 meat	1 meat	1 fruit
1 dairy	1 dairy	3 grains	1 grain
2 fruits	1 grain	3 vegetables	1 nuts
1 fat	1 vegetable	1½ fat servings	
1 fat	1 fruit	1 fruit	

TABLE 9-4   An Example of a 2,000-Calorie DASH Meal Plan

Breakfast	Lunch	Dinner	Snack
1 cup corn flakes	2 ounces chicken	3 ounces salmon	1 medium apple
1 cup 1% milk	½ ounce low-fat cheddar	1 cup rice	1 slice wheat bread
1 banana	1 pita bread	1 cup squash	⅓ cup pecans
1 slice wheat toast	1 teaspoon margarine	1 cup spinach	
1 tablespoon jam	1 cup raw carrots	1 tablespoon light Italian dressing	
6 ounces apple juice	1 orange	1½ ounces low-fat Jack cheese	
1 teaspoon margarine			

TABLE 9-5   Another Example of a 2,000-Calorie DASH Meal Plan

Breakfast	Lunch	Dinner	Snack
1 cup prune juice	2 ounces lean beef	3 ounces trout	1 orange
1 cup oatmeal	1 teaspoon barbecue sauce	1 cup brown rice	1 ounce dried fruit
1 slice whole wheat bread	1 roll	1 cup three-bean salad	2 tablespoons sunflower seeds
1 teaspoon margarine	1 cup boiled potatoes	1 tablespoon low-fat dressing	
1 cup 1% milk	¼ cup low-fat cheddar	1½-ounce corn muffin	
1 banana	1 cup lettuce salad	1 teaspoon margarine	
1 cup cranberry juice	1 tablespoon low-fat dressing	1 cup spinach	

Helpful hints and resources

TIP

The following suggestions can help you as you begin to incorporate this nutrition plan into your daily life:

>> Don't try to change all at once. Gradually eat less meat and more fruits and vegetables.

>> Increase your fruit and vegetable servings by having two at each meal and two for a snack.

>> If you're lactose intolerant, try lactose-free milk.

>> Reduce your fat consumption so you're eating half your normal intake; emphasize vegetable fats over animal fats.

>> Avoid soda, alcohol, and other sugar-sweetened drinks.

>> Have fruit for dessert.

>> Instead of meat, fish, or poultry, make grains (like pasta and rice), beans, and vegetables the center of the meal.

TIP

An informative website about the DASH diet is www.nhlbi.nih.gov/education/dash-eating-plan. Other valuable sources of information about DASH include the following:

>> **DASH Diet Eating Plan:** https://dashdiet.org

>> **DASH Diet Recipes:** www.mayoclinic.org/healthy-lifestyle/recipes/dash-diet-recipes/rcs-20077146

Reducing your salt consumption with DASH

Chapter 10 does a deep dive on salt and high blood pressure, but the bottom line is this: The less salt in your diet, the lower your blood pressure. If you want to combine DASH with a low-salt diet, here are some suggestions:

>> Buy products that have *reduced sodium* or *no salt added* on their labels.

>> Use herbs, spices, a little wine, lemon, lime, or vinegar instead of salt to flavor your food.

>> Leave the saltshaker in the kitchen, away from the table, to help you fight the urge to add more salt when eating. Out of sight, out of mind!

>> Emphasize eating more unprocessed foods. Mother Nature knows what she's doing!

- » Avoid high-salt condiments like soy sauce, teriyaki sauce, and monosodium glutamate (MSG).

- » Reduce your intake of foods in brine and mustard, salt-cured foods, horseradish, ketchup, and Worcestershire sauce.

- » Eat fruits and vegetables for snacks instead of salty snack foods.

- » Avoid salty foods when eating out.

TIP

Just because you're following a DASH nutrition plan doesn't mean you can't eat out. It just means you need to plan ahead. The menus of many restaurants are available online, allowing you to figure out what you're going to eat.

Maximizing the Mediterranean Diet to Lower Your Blood Pressure

In addition to the DASH diet, another well-studied nutrition plan is the Mediterranean diet. People who live in countries near the Mediterranean Sea, including Spain, France, Italy, and Greece, have a lower mortality from cardiovascular disease when compared to other countries, and their diet is one reason way. The Mediterranean diet has many beneficial effects — it helps delay or even prevent cardiovascular disease, reduces cancer risk, decreases inflammation, reduces the risk of metabolic syndrome (see "Losing Weight with Nutrition," later in this chapter), and reduces blood pressure.

The Mediterranean diet is similar in many respects to DASH. It's rich in fruits and vegetables, as well as whole grains. Plus, the Mediterranean diet includes fish, poultry, lean meat, and seafood, but the core focus of the diet is on whole grains, fruits, and vegetables. A staple of the Mediterranean diet is olive oil and other unsaturated fats.

TECHNICAL
STUFF

The increased omega-3 fish oil content of the Mediterranean diet has significant anti-inflammatory components that reduce markers of inflammation, such as C-reactive protein (CRP).

A Mediterranean diet is very beneficial for lowering high blood pressure. In one study that looked at more than 1,100 individuals, there was a reduction in the systolic blood pressure of 9 points in males and 3 points in females. The study also noted improvement in arterial stiffness. In a review of several clinical trials, the Mediterranean diet was shown to be effective in lowering blood pressure. The longer a person maintained this nutrition plan, the more sustained the decreased effect on blood pressure was.

Seeing the Value of a Plant-Based Diet Plan

DASH and the Mediterranean diet aren't the only healthy eating plans out there. Whatever you choose, consider a nutrition program in which a plant-based program is at its core. The advantages of a plant-based nutrition program are that you can eat all the green leafy vegetables you want, and you aren't consuming a lot of calories.

TIP

One plant-based nutrition plan that's successful in helping people to improve their health, lower their blood pressure, and lose weight is the Nutritarian diet. Founded by Dr. Joel Fuhrman, this nutrition plan recommends the consumption of a nutrient-based plan. Many people have been helped by incorporating this nutrition plan in their daily lives. For more information, head to www.drfurhman.com/blog/210/beginners-guide.

Losing Weight with Nutrition

Metabolic syndrome isn't so much a disease as a collection of risk factors that increase your risk for diabetes and cardiovascular disease. These risk factors include the following:

>> High blood pressure

>> High triglycerides and low high density lipoprotein (HDL)

>> Increased waist circumference

>> *Hyperinsulinemia* (high levels of insulin in the body)

>> Impaired fasting blood glucose (blood glucose levels between 100 and 125 mg/dL)

Metabolic syndrome is associated with higher levels of total body inflammation and overlaps with increased BMI (in which you're classified as overweight or obese).

TIP

I look at BMI as well as waist circumference in the context of metabolic syndrome and overall health. BMI is an important component, but it isn't the only component. My own discussions with patients have been on improving health not losing weight.

REMEMBER

Lowering high blood pressure is important, but you can't stop there. Nutrition is key not only in lowering your blood pressure, but also in lowering inflammation, preventing or reversing metabolic syndrome, reducing cardiovascular risk, and preventing the development of end organ complications related to high blood pressure (see Part 2).

TIP

To get a better sense of the effect of weight on blood pressure, note that for every 2.2 pounds of weight you lose, your systolic blood pressure drops by 1 mm Hg and your diastolic blood pressure drops by 1 mm Hg. In other words, if your blood pressure has been 135/85 and you lose 11 pounds, your blood pressure would fall to 130/80.

Calculating your ideal weight

Many health-care providers use an ideal weight just as a baseline in order to approximate how much weight you may need to lose to help improve your blood pressure and overall health.

The BMI is a measurement used to help determine if someone is underweight, overweight, or obese. By definition, a BMI of 18.5 to 249.9 is normal, a BMI of 25 to 29.9 is overweight, and a BMI of 30 or greater is obese. You can find your BMI by going to www.nhlbi.nih.gov/health/educational/lose_wt/BMI/bmicalc. htm or using Table 9-6 (just find your height in the left-hand column and move along that row until you reach your approximate weight — your BMI is at the top of that column).

REMEMBER

BMI is important, but it isn't the only thing that matters. Everyone is built differently, and we all have different body types. If you have questions about BMI and your "ideal" weight, talk with your doctor.

Determining your daily caloric needs

Caloric needs are different depending on age, sex, and level of activity. For example, if a woman is pregnant or breastfeeding, she needs more calories. But if a person is trying to lose weight, they need to reduce calories. When you know the appropriate weight for your height, you can determine the number of daily calories to either maintain or reduce your present weight. Consider working with a dietitian to make sure you're getting the right nutrients while staying within your daily caloric limits.

TABLE 9-6 **Body Mass Index Chart**

Height	19	20	21	22	23	24	25	26	27	28	29	30	35	40
	Body Weight (in Pounds)													
4'10"	91	96	100	105	110	115	119	124	129	134	138	143	167	191
4'11"	94	99	104	109	114	119	124	128	133	138	143	148	173	198
5'	97	102	107	112	118	123	128	133	138	143	148	153	179	204
5'1"	100	106	111	116	122	127	132	137	143	148	153	158	185	211
5'2"	104	109	115	120	126	131	136	142	147	153	158	164	191	218
5'3"	107	113	118	124	130	135	141	146	152	158	163	169	197	225
5'4"	110	116	122	128	134	140	145	151	157	163	169	174	204	232
5'5"	114	120	126	132	138	144	150	156	162	168	174	180	210	240
5'6"	118	124	130	136	142	148	155	161	167	173	179	186	216	247
5'7"	121	127	134	140	146	153	159	166	172	178	185	191	223	255
5'8"	125	131	138	144	151	158	164	171	177	184	190	197	230	262
5'9"	128	135	142	149	155	162	169	176	182	189	196	203	236	270
5'10"	132	139	146	153	160	167	174	181	188	195	202	207	243	278
5'11"	136	143	150	157	165	172	179	186	193	200	208	215	250	286
6'	140	147	154	162	169	177	184	191	199	206	213	221	258	294
6'1"	144	151	159	166	174	182	189	197	204	212	219	227	265	302
6'2"	148	155	163	171	179	186	194	202	210	218	225	233	272	311
6'3"	152	160	168	176	184	192	200	208	216	224	232	240	279	319
6'4"	156	164	172	180	189	197	205	213	221	230	238	246	287	328

REMEMBER

One pound of fat contains 3,500 calories. To lose a pound of fat, therefore, you must eat 3,500 calories less than you need. You can do this a couple of ways:

>> By reducing your daily intake 500 calories for seven days

>> By doing 200 calories of exercise per day (see Chapter 12) and reducing your diet by only 300 calories per day

LOWERING YOUR WAIST CIRCUMFERENCE

Increased waist circumference is a risk factor for the development of heart disease, worsening high blood pressure, and diabetes. A waist circumference more than 40 inches in men and more than 35 inches in women puts you at high risk for the development of heart disease and diabetes.

When you see your health-care provider in the office, they should record your blood pressure, BMI, and waist measurement.

To reduce your waist circumference, get at least 30 minutes of aerobic exercise a day (see Chapter 12), do strength training two or three times a week (see Chapter 12), stick to a healthy diet (like the ones I cover in this chapter), get seven to nine hours of sleep a night, and reduce stress by doing simple activities like meditation or yoga.

For most people, a combination of diet and exercise seems to work much better than diet alone.

REMEMBER

You don't have to lose weight all the way down to your appropriate range to benefit from weight loss. A loss of 5 percent to 10 percent of your current weight brings important benefits in terms of lowering blood pressure, improving triglycerides, and lowering blood glucose.

TECHNICAL STUFF

Understanding caloric intake and what your body needs calorie-wise is important. That said, the effect of hyperinsulinemia, another aspect of metabolic syndrome, can really affect a person's ability to lose weight. Insulin is a hormone that is produced by the pancreas in response to carbohydrate intake. Insulin is a "storage" hormone, meaning it promotes the body's storage of fat. This is why it can be difficult to lose weight even if you're consuming the right amount of calories — the high insulin levels are going to prevent you from losing weight. This is why a holistic approach is needed for the treatment of high blood pressure — you shouldn't rely on weight loss alone.

Adjusting your DASH nutrition plan

When you know your daily caloric goal, you can go back to "Getting with the program," earlier in this chapter, and subtract or add servings appropriately. To figure out the DASH program at a lower caloric range without the assistance of a dietitian, Table 9-7 shows the breakdown of servings for 2,000-, 1,800-, and 1,500-calorie DASH programs.

TABLE 9-7

Daily Servings Comparison for 2,000-, 1,800-, and 1,500-Calorie DASH

Food Group	2,000 Calories	1,800 Calories	1,500 Calories
Grains	8 per day	8 per day	5½ per day
Vegetables	4 per day	4 per day	4 per day
Fruits	5 per day	4 per day	4 per day
Dairy	3 per day	3 per day	3 per day
Meats and fish	2 per day	1¾ per day	1¾ per day
Fats and oils	2½ per day	2½ per day	1½ per day
Nuts and seeds	1 per day	1 per day	¾ per day
Sweets	5 per week	3 per week	2 per week

TIP

One effective way to meet your weight-loss goal is the half-portion plan. If you're eating at home, simply cut the portion in half and save the other half for another meal. If you're eating out, consider sharing an entree with someone else. Many restaurants serve much more food than anyone should eat at one meal. Take advantage of it!

TIP

If you're following the DASH diet, you can significantly reduce calories with some simple substitutions:

>> Use fat-free or low-fat condiments.

>> Cut the amount of oil or dressing in half. ***Remember:*** Oil has a lot of calories!

>> Drink low-fat milk.

>> Check labels for added sugar.

>> Avoid fruits canned in sugary syrup.

>> Add fruit to plain yogurt.

>> Snack on carrot sticks, celery sticks, plain popcorn, or rice cakes.

>> Avoid caloric drinks; stick to water with lemon or lime.

Consulting with a Nutritionist

A nutritionist can be a tremendous source of information on all aspects of nutrition. They can help you determine your correct weight and the ideal number of calories you should eat per day to reach that weight. Your health-care provider or local hospital can provide the name of a reputable nutritionist or dietitian.

Nutrition is an important and underemphasized aspect of high blood pressure and health. In my opinion, everyone should have an annual visit with a nutritionist. Nutrition is too important not to. Proper nutrition can help you improve chronic medical conditions, lower blood pressure, and improve your total body health. Having an expert by your side can make all the difference.

Chapter **10**

Keeping Salt and Sugar Out of Your Diet

A cornerstone in the treatment of high blood pressure has been limiting the amount of salt you're consuming on a daily basis. The effects of high blood pressure medications are enhanced when you restrict the amount of salt you take in. In addition to limiting your intake of salt, an additional component of treating high blood pressure is limiting your sugar intake.

In this chapter, you read about the effects of salt and sugar on high blood pressure. I explain how you can decrease the amount of salt in your food, what foods are low or high in salt, and what's in a low-salt diet. I also outline the effects of sugar on high blood pressure. You can't control your genetics or your age, but you *can* control what you eat, and salt and sugar are two big factors that deserve your attention.

Making the Connection between Salt and High Blood Pressure

Sodium is necessary for life — you can't live without it. Sodium helps maintain your blood's water content, balances the acids and bases in your blood, and is necessary for the electrical charges in your nerves that move your muscles.

One of the main functions of the kidneys is elimination of excess sodium that the body doesn't need. If you consume more sodium than your body needs, your blood pressure increases and the kidneys have to filter and eliminate more sodium. Over time, that increased blood pressure increases the stress on your cardiovascular system, which is one important aspect in the development of heart disease.

TECHNICAL STUFF

You may be reading this and asking yourself, "What's the difference between salt and sodium?" Although those terms are often used interchangeably, there is a subtle difference. Sodium makes up about 40 percent of salt; the other 60 percent is chloride. One teaspoon of salt is the equivalent of 2,300 mg (or about 1 teaspoon) of sodium.

Proving the connection between sodium and high blood pressure

In the early 20th century, the first experiments on the connection between salt and blood pressure showed that blood pressure improved as the consumption of salt was reduced. You can find these studies in the *Archives of General Medicine* (February 1904).

A low-salt diet reduced blood pressure in half of the patients who had high blood pressure. In the rest of the patients, changes may have been irreversible (in other words, the blood pressure no longer responded to salt deprivation alone), or some patients may not have been as salt sensitive (I discuss salt sensitivity later in this chapter).

In the *American Journal of Medicine* (March 1948), a study established without a doubt that salt restriction lowers blood pressure. Shortly afterward, however, the first *diuretics* (blood pressure drugs that increase salt and water excretion; see Chapter 13) came on the market. As a result, salt restriction as a means of lowering blood pressure fell out of favor. But we know now that salt restriction enhances the blood-pressure-lowering effects of diuretics as well as the blood-pressure-lowering effects of other medications.

In 1988, the Intersalt Study, a huge study of more than 10,000 people from many nations, showed that salt intake is directly related to the rise of both systolic and diastolic blood pressures with age (see Chapter 2 for more about these types of blood pressure). The researchers concluded that reducing salt intake by 1 teaspoon daily from age 25 to age 55 can reduce blood pressure by 9 mm Hg. *Note:* People who lived where salt consumption was lowest had no increase in blood pressure with age.

LOOKING AT THE ROLE OF POTASSIUM

Your body is geared toward balance, and it's no difference when it comes to electrolytes and blood pressure. Limiting your intake of sodium is really important, but so is increasing your consumption of potassium. A 2021 study from the *Journal of Clinical Hypertension* looked at the ratio of sodium to potassium consumption and found that people with high blood pressure had a high sodium intake a low potassium intake. If you can change your sodium-to-potassium ratio — in other words, decrease your sodium intake while increasing your potassium intake — you'll help improve your blood pressure.

Here's the good news: A nutrition plan low in sodium and high in fruits and vegetables will also be high in potassium.

Some medical conditions (such as chronic kidney disease and diabetes) and some medications (like ACE inhibitors — see Chapter 13) may limit the amount of potassium you can consume, and you may have to adjust your content of high-potassium foods.

Note: Pay attention to the ingredients in salt substitutes. Many contain potassium chloride. While potassium consumption can lower blood pressure, the excess potassium in the salt substitute can raise your potassium levels to very high levels, especially if you treat your salt substitute like a salt shaker. If your body's potassium levels get too high, it can have an adverse effect on your heart. Talk with your health-care provider before using any salt substitute.

Looking at salt sensitivity

Limiting your intake of sodium is an important aspect of treatment for high blood pressure, but if you have salt sensitivity, sodium restriction takes on even more importance. More than 50 percent of people with high blood pressure are likely salt sensitive. Individuals who may be more at risk for developing salt sensitivity include

>> People over the age of 65

>> People who are overweight

>> People with diabetes

>> People with chronic kidney disease

>> African Americans

>> Women

REMEMBER

Reduce your salt intake whether you're salt sensitive or not because

>> If you're salt sensitive, the reduction really helps to reduce your blood pressure.

>> If you're not salt sensitive, the reduced salt intake can also help to reduce your blood pressure, as well as improve the blood-pressure-lowering effects of medications that you're taking.

Lowering your salt intake

Reading labels is important in knowing the salt content of foods that you're eating. A lot of salt is used in the processing of foods, so it isn't surprising that highly processed foods can contain a lot of salt.

REMEMBER

To reduce the salt content in your diet, you have to switch from processed foods to fresh foods such as fruits and vegetables.

Reading food labels

REMEMBER

The U.S. Food and Drug Administration (FDA) has guidelines for food companies regarding a product's sodium content description. Keep these terms in mind when reading food labels, and make a point of buying low-sodium foods on your next trip to the grocery store:

>> **Low sodium** means less than 140 mg of sodium per serving.

>> **Very low sodium** means less than 35 mg of sodium per serving.

>> **Sodium free** means less than 5 mg of sodium per serving.

>> **Reduced sodium** means 25 percent less sodium than the original food item.

>> **Light in sodium** means 50 percent less sodium than the original food item.

>> **Unsalted, no salt added, and without added salt** mean absolutely no salt has been added to a food that's normally processed with salt.

TIP

Take the time to also read the ingredients section on food items. Really look at anything marked "sodium." One example is the food additive monosodium glutamate (MSG). The more informed you are as a consumer, the better food choices you'll make.

Avoiding high-salt foods

Here's a list of processed foods that have a high sodium content. Avoid eating these foods as much as possible:

>> Anchovies

>> Bacon

>> Bouillon cubes

>> Canned soups

>> Canned tuna

>> Canned vegetables

>> Cheese

>> Cold cuts

>> Condiments

>> Cooking sauce (prepared high-sodium sauce)

>> Cottage cheese

>> Croutons

>> Gravy

>> Ham

>> Hot dogs

>> Olives

>> Pickles

>> Salad dressing

>> Salsa

>> Sausage

>> Sea salt

>> Soy sauce

>> Spaghetti sauce

>> Sweet-and-sour sauce

>> Tomato or vegetable juice

>> Tomato sauce

Going on a low-salt diet

TIP

Besides avoiding high-salt foods, you can make a few other changes to lower your salt intake:

>> Cook with herbs, spices, fruit juices, and vinegars, instead of salt, to add flavor.

>> Eat fresh vegetables.

>> Keep the saltshaker in the kitchen cupboard instead of at the table, where it's so easy to use.

>> Use less salt than the recipe calls for.

>> Select low-salt canned foods or rinse the food with water after removing it from the can.

>> Opt for low-salt frozen dinners.

>> Use high-salt condiments like ketchup and mustard sparingly.

>> Snack on fresh fruits instead of salted crackers or chips.

>> When eating out, ask that your food be prepared with only a little salt. Request your salad dressing on the side so you can control the amount.

WARNING

Be careful of salt substitutes because some contain sodium. You may end up eating so much of the substitute to get that salty taste that your total sodium intake is just as high as it would be if you were using salt. Check the label!

COMBINING A LOW-SALT DIET WITH DASH

Chapter 9 explains the DASH nutritional program in detail. Combine DASH with a low-salt diet to get the maximum blood-pressure-lowering effect. Some recommendations for the various food groups in DASH are as follows:

- **Grains:** Check the salt content of all prepared grain foods, and keep the sodium less than 180 mg in each serving. Avoid any salted grain foods such as salted popcorn.

- **Fruits:** Avoid dried fruits with salt.

- **Vegetables:** Eat fresh vegetables and read the label on prepared vegetables.

- **Meats:** Eat fresh meats, fish, and poultry; avoid salt-cured products.

- **Dairy products:** Avoid products with more than 180 mg of sodium per serving.

- **Fats:** Avoid high-salt salad dressings and salted butter.

- **Nuts and seeds:** Avoid salted varieties.

- **Sweets:** Avoid sweets that contain more than 180 mg of sodium per serving.

Connecting Sugar and High Blood Pressure: The Role of Insulin

You probably knew about the connection between salt and high blood pressure, but you may not have known about the role of sugar in high blood pressure.

All sugar is carbohydrate, but there are simple carbohydrates and complex carbohydrates:

>> **Simple carbohydrates:** Simple carbohydrates include glucose, fructose, and sucrose, and they have a tendency to really affect insulin levels, causing weight gain, fat deposits, and high blood pressure. Foods that fall into this category include white bread, white pasta, sugary breakfast cereals, cake, candy, and so on.

>> **Complex carbohydrates:** Complex carbohydrates take longer to digest, and because of this, your body's glucose level rises more slowly, which is less likely to trigger an abrupt increase in insulin. Foods that fall into this category include whole grains (like brown rice, oats, and quinoa), lentils, and beans.

The effect of sugar consumption on high blood pressure is multifaceted. First, excess sugar consumption is associated with weight gain and obesity, which is a risk factor for high blood pressure. But high insulin levels may contribute to high blood pressure, too.

With consumption of any type of sugar, the common denominator is the stimulation of insulin by the body. Think of insulin as a storage hormone — it's stimulated by glucose and sugar intake, and it causes your body to store the calories from the food you've consumed. Very high insulin levels in the body can stimulate the development of high blood pressure. People with both high insulin levels in the body (also referred to as *hyperinsulinemia*) and insulin resistance often have higher blood pressure than people with lower insulin levels do.

WARNING

Avoid anything that is made with fructose or high-fructose corn syrup. Fructose is processed by the body a little differently than other sugars. It increases the risk of weight gain and fat deposits in the body. It also increases the formation of uric acid, which is thought to have a role in insulin resistance and high blood pressure. Plus, it increases the risk of developing fatty liver disease, metabolic syndrome (see the nearby sidebar), and obesity. High-fructose corn syrup is found in sugary soft drinks, ice cream, fast foods, and many other foods — read the labels!

REDUCING YOUR RISK OF METABOLIC SYNDROME AND DIABETES

Metabolic syndrome is a group of conditions:

- Increased blood pressure

- Increased waist circumference

- Increased triglyceride levels (usually more than 150 mg/dL)

- Low high-density lipoprotein (HDL) levels (usually less than 40 mg/dL)

- Impaired fasting glucose levels (usually between 100 and 125 mg/dL)

You only need three out of these five criteria to be diagnosed with metabolic syndrome. And metabolic syndrome increases your risk of developing diabetes, heart disease, and worsening high blood pressure. What can you do about this? Adopt a DASH nutrition plan or a plant-based nutrition plan (see Chapter 9) and get more exercise (see Chapter 12).

If you have metabolic syndrome or you've been told you have impaired fasting glucose (often referred to as prediabetes) or even diabetes, you need to be aware of the glycemic index, which is a measure of a food's ability to raise glucose levels. The glycemic index is based on a scale from 0 to 100 — the higher the food's glycemic index, the more it raises a person's glucose levels.

Very sweet fruits such as watermelon have a high glycemic index. Other fruits, such as bananas and raisins, have a moderate to high glycemic index. Be sure to choose fruit with a lower glycemic index, including berries, apples, and cherries. To find the glycemic index of any food, search the web for "glycemic index of" and the name of the food (for example, "glycemic index of bananas").

Two other important things you can do to reduce your risk of metabolic syndrome is limit your sodium intake and avoiding foods and drinks with high-fructose corn syrup.

Chapter **11**

Avoiding Tobacco, Alcohol, and Caffeine

When it comes to your blood pressure, the 80/20 rule applies: Eighty percent of the consequences of any action come from 20 percent of the things you do or don't do. Tobacco, alcohol, and caffeine are all part of that 20 percent. If you can limit or quit these things, you can reduce your blood pressure and begin to feel great!

Quitting or reducing your consumption of any of these substances isn't easy. But nothing you do for your health can make a greater difference than cutting out tobacco and significantly reducing your consumption of alcohol and caffeine.

This chapter explores each of these substances in greater detail, including how they affect your blood pressure and how reducing your consumption of them can help lower your blood pressure and make your mind and body healthier in the process.

TIP

Tobacco, alcohol, and caffeine often go hand in hand. It isn't uncommon, for example, for someone to have a cigarette with their morning coffee. Reducing or eliminating your consumption of coffee might help you quit smoking, or vice versa.

Playing with Fire: Tobacco and High Blood Pressure

If you play with fire, you run the risk of getting burned. If you smoke, you run the risk of getting burned inside and out. Whether tobacco is smoked, chewed, or consumed by any other means, the nicotine in tobacco raises your blood pressure. The more you smoke, the higher the nicotine level in your blood and the higher your blood pressure. To a large extent, this effect accounts for the significantly increased risk of stroke (see Chapter 7), heart disease (see Chapter 5), and pain in the legs due to poor circulation among people who smoke.

Nicotine raises your blood pressure by constricting or narrowing your blood vessels. The oxygen content in your blood decreases as the nicotine directly stimulates the production of *epinephrine* (also known as *adrenaline*, a hormone that raises blood pressure) in the adrenal gland.

Numerous studies have shown that smoking and chewing tobacco raise blood pressure and that when you stop using tobacco products, your blood pressure falls. One study in the *Journal of Hypertension* (March 2007) comes from China. For ten years, researchers followed 10,525 men and women who did not initially have high blood pressure. At the end of the study, key predictors of future high blood pressure included age, weight, excess alcohol, and cigarette smoking.

REMEMBER

Although nicotine is what increases blood pressure, other substances in cigarettes have cancer-causing effects. Your health will benefit health from quitting smoking, no matter your age or physical condition.

Examining the extent of the problem

According to the U.S. Centers for Disease Control and Prevention (CDC), in 2021 approximately 28 million adults in the United States smoked cigarettes. Worldwide, as of 2022, there are more than 1.1 *billion* smokers. In the United States, 13 percent of white adults, 12 percent of Black adults, 8 percent of Hispanic adults, and approximately 5 percent of all Asian adults smoke. And as we all know, smoking isn't just limited to adults: According to the CDC, every day approximately 2,000 adolescents will smoke their first cigarette and about 300 of those people will continue to smoke daily.

These statistics only deal with regular cigarette smoking. What about electronic cigarettes or vaping? According to the CDC, more than 2.5 million middle and high school students reported using e-cigarettes in 2022. This includes about 14 percent of high school students and about 3 percent of middle school students.

The harmful effects of nicotine on blood pressure aren't limited to traditional cigarettes. E-cigarettes are associated with high blood pressure, as well as increased cardiovascular risk.

Understanding the consequences of tobacco use

In addition to its effects on blood pressure, tobacco use has other health consequences, including the following:

>> The risk of lung cancer is significantly higher among smokers than nonsmokers.

>> Mouth and throat cancer, as well as bladder cancer, are more common among smokers than among nonsmokers. Smoking is likely to increase the risk of other forms of cancer as well.

>> The risk of heart disease is higher among smokers than among nonsmokers. This risk is significant even if you don't have high blood pressure.

>> The risk of stroke is higher in smokers than it is in nonsmokers.

>> The risk of lung disease, including chronic obstructive pulmonary disease (COPD), is a consequence of long-term smoking.

>> Lung growth rate is decreased among adolescents who smoke.

>> Smoking reduces bone density and increases the risk of fractures, especially in older women.

>> Tobacco dries and wrinkles the skin and yellows your teeth, fingers, and fingernails.

>> A correlation exists between smoking and depression.

Given the multiple ways that smoking can adversely affect your health, if you are not a smoker, don't start. If you are a smoker, do everything you can to quit.

Reducing your exposure to secondhand smoke

Secondhand smoke (also referred to as *passive smoking*) is inhaled from someone else's cigarette, and it's a risk to anyone who's exposed to it. Daily exposure to secondhand smoke is a risk factor for high blood pressure. Secondhand smoke also increases the risk of heart disease — the risk is thought to be just as significant as if you were the one smoking.

According to data from the CDC, more than 41,000 people die every year due to secondhand smoke. Approximately 7,300 of these deaths are due to lung cancer and about 34,000 of these deaths are due to heart disease.

TIP

Don't become a victim of secondhand smoke. Follow these guidelines:

>> **Don't allow anyone to smoke in your home or car.** If someone in your household smokes, ask them to do so outside and away from the house.

>> **Never smoke with children around.**

>> **If you can't avoid your exposure to secondhand smoke, improve ventilation by opening windows and/or using an air purifier.**

Avoiding all forms of tobacco

Smokeless tobacco is tobacco that you don't actually smoke. Types of smokeless tobacco include

>> **Snuff:** Snuff comes in dried and moist forms. The dried form of snuff is placed in the nostrils; the moist form of snuff is placed between the cheek and the gum.

>> **Chewing tobacco:** Chewing tobacco is a wad of tobacco placed inside the cheek and chewed on to extract the juices, which are spit out. You may have seen baseball players chewing tobacco and spitting out the juice.

Smokeless tobacco provides at least twice as much nicotine as cigarettes. Eight to ten chews daily is the equivalent of smoking 40 cigarettes when it comes to the amount of nicotine. So, smokeless tobacco damages the heart and blood vessels over the long term, and it has greater and longer effects on blood pressure than cigarettes do. Plus, smokeless tobacco increases the risk of developing head and neck cancer.

REMEMBER

Smokeless tobacco is not an alternative to cigarette smoking, and it can't help you quit smoking. In fact, smokeless tobacco:

>> Is very addictive

>> Doesn't eliminate nicotine cravings

>> Can discolor your teeth and sour your breath

>> Increases the risk of developing cancer in your throat, voice box, and esophagus

Quitting tobacco successfully

Quitting tobacco is difficult but not impossible. There are more tools available today to help you quit than ever before. No one way works for all people. If one method doesn't work, try another. Eventually, if you keep at it, you'll succeed!

In the following sections, I walk you through the basics of quitting tobacco, but check out *Quitting Smoking & Vaping For Dummies*, by Charles H. Elliot and Laura L. Smith (published by Wiley), for a lot more information.

Keys to quitting

There are five steps to quitting tobacco. If you relapse, begin again with Step 1.

1. Prepare yourself.

Set a quit date and make it special. After all, this is the first day of the rest of your new life!

Leading up to your big day:

- Make a list of reasons to quit and post it on your refrigerator.
- Improve your fitness, which makes any significant change easier to manage. You can do something as simple as walking 30 minutes a day.
- Cut back on your caffeine consumption. This will help you sleep after you quit smoking.
- Satisfy your hunger with low-calorie beverages or snacks.
- Incorporate meditation or another mindfulness-based activity (like yoga) into your daily routine as a stress reliever. You can even do some deep breathing at your desk instead of taking a smoke break.

2. Benefit from the support of friends and loved ones.

Let everyone know you're quitting and ask for help, especially by not smoking in your presence. Even better, ask them to stop *with* you.

Consider incorporating individual or group counseling for additional support. This may mean talking to someone as needed when you're trying to quit. Check with your health-care provider for options in your area.

3. Use new skills to handle problems that arise.

Find enjoyable distractions (like exercising, reading a good book, or watching a good movie) that substitute for the urge to smoke.

Stop activities that you used to combine with smoking (like drinking coffee first thing in the morning, having a nightcap, or whatever you know to be your smoking trigger).

Change your routine to emphasize this change in lifestyle. For example, go for a short walk first thing in the morning instead of lighting up.

Before you stop:

- Switch to a brand that you don't like that's low in nicotine.
- Smoke only half the cigarette.
- Limit yourself to an increasingly smaller fixed number of cigarettes daily.
- Drink plenty of noncaloric fluids such as water.

4. **Make use of the medications that have proven to be effective in helping people quit.**

   Ask your doctor about nicotine replacement therapy and smoking cessation aids.

5. **Prepare for relapses.**

   Everyone who has successfully quit smoking has probably done it on the second, third, or fourth try. Giving yourself a break when this happens means giving yourself another chance to succeed. A relapse often occurs within the first three months. You can avoid situations most likely to trigger a relapse by doing the following:

   - Try not to consume alcohol, which can lessen your control and increase your desire for a cigarette.
   - Try to avoid being around people who smoke. It'll be hard to quit if you're standing outside talking to smokers as they light up.
   - If you gain weight, don't start smoking again to try to lose it. Instead, try adding some more exercise to your daily routine.
   - Do your best not to treat your nervousness, depression, or anxiety with a cigarette.

TIP

If you relapse, begin the process of quitting again as soon as possible. The less you smoke before beginning again, the easier it will be to quit. Try to recognize the situations that affected your ability to successfully quit on your previous attempts and avoid them the next time around.

Effective methods of quitting

Two effective methods for quitting smoking are nicotine replacement therapy and smoking cessation aids. You can buy some methods over the counter; others require a prescription from your doctor.

REMEMBER

Talk with your health-care provider before beginning any of these interventions especially if you have high blood pressure or other health conditions.

NICOTINE-REPLACEMENT THERAPY

The point of nicotine replacement therapy is to deliver small doses of nicotine to reduce the withdrawal symptoms. The therapy comes in five forms:

>> **Nicotine gum:** Available over the counter, nicotine gum comes in 2-mg and 4-mg strengths. As you chew, nicotine is released and absorbed through the lining of your mouth. By reducing the number of pieces each day, you reach a day when you need none.

>> **Nicotine lozenges:** Available over the counter, nicotine lozenges come in 2-mg and 4-mg doses. As you suck on the lozenge, nicotine is released and absorbed through the lining of your mouth.

>> **Nicotine patches:** Available over the counter and by prescription, the nicotine patches come in three strengths: 7 mg, 14 mg, and 21 mg. You apply the patch to your skin (usually your upper arm, chest, or back), and nicotine is gradually released and absorbed through the skin. You typically start with the highest strength and work your way down to the lowest strength.

>> *Note:* People with allergies to adhesives may have trouble wearing a nicotine patch. Combining the gum or lozenges with the patches may work better than either alone, but be sure to get your doctor's approval before using both treatments together.

>> **Nicotine nasal spray:** Available by prescription only, you use the spray whenever you have the urge to smoke. People with a sinus condition typically find it difficult to use.

>> **Nicotine inhalers:** Available by prescription, inhalers deliver nicotine in a vapor into the mouth, where it's absorbed through the lining of the mouth. The inhalant may irritate the mouth and throat.

WARNING

If you have high blood pressure associated with nicotine intake, plan to use this therapy as short a time as possible because nicotine in this form still raises your blood pressure.

SMOKING-CESSATION AIDS

The following smoking-cessation aids don't contain nicotine, but they do decrease withdrawal symptoms. New preparations seem to appear almost daily. Some examples include the following:

>> **Bupropion SR (trade name: Zyban):** Available by prescription, Zyban acts to disrupt the addictive power of nicotine. At a dose of 150 mg taken twice a day, it has been proven effective in large studies of smokers.

TIP

A combination of bupropion and nicotine-replacement therapy (see the preceding section) accomplished a much higher rate of quitting than either one did alone.

>> **Varenicline (trade name: Chantix):** Available by prescription, Chantix acts within the brain to diminish the high from smoking and decrease withdrawal symptoms. The dose is 1 mg taken twice a day.

Tapping into resources

You can find all kinds of helpful resources on the internet to help you on your journey to quit tobacco. Here are some examples:

>> **Agency for Healthcare Research and Quality** (www.ahrq.gov): The Agency for Healthcare Research and Quality has smoking cessation guidelines and other materials for both health-care professionals and the general public.

>> **American Cancer Society** (www.cancer.org): The American Cancer Society has a lot of information on quitting smoking, as well as links to other resources.

>> **American Lung Association** (www.lung.org): The American Lung Association is another informative source to help you stop smoking.

>> **Centers for Disease Control and Prevention** (www.cdc.gov/tobacco): The CDC website has a database of smoking and health-related materials. You can also call 800-232-4636 for more information.

>> **Nicotine Anonymous** (www.nicotine-anonymous.org): Nicotine Anonymous is a 12-step program. To find out more, visit the website or call 415-750-0328.

Linking Alcohol to High Blood Pressure

Simply put, alcohol raises blood pressure. When individuals who do not normally drink *do* consume alcohol, their blood pressure rises, and when individuals with significant alcohol use *stop* drinking, their blood pressure lowers. Chronic alcohol use over time increases blood pressure.

WARNING

Not that long ago, a daily glass of red wine was touted as having cardiovascular benefits. But today we know that *any* amount of daily alcohol consumption has risks, and the risks outweigh the benefits.

If your drinking has been moderate to heavy on a daily basis, and you abruptly stop drinking, it may cause a dangerous increase in your blood pressure. If you're thinking about quitting alcohol, talk with your health-care provider. You should quit with their supervision.

Consuming large quantities of alcohol in one sitting (or standing, depending on the location!) also raises blood pressure and can have a rapid toxic effect on the heart. This effect is seen often during the holidays when people may drink to excess, often while eating a lot of high-sodium foods. If you also have a cigarette in the midst of all this fun, that can raise your blood pressure even more. Be careful, especially over the holidays.

Long-term alcohol use increases the risk of developing *cirrhosis* (scarring) of the liver. It's also associated with the development of high blood pressure. Other long-term of consequences of alcohol use include the following:

>> Decreased ability to perform reliably complex tasks, like driving;

>> Decreased attention span and short-term memory

>> Impaired motor coordination

>> Difficulty walking

>> Damage to the nerves in the hands and feet (known as *peripheral neuropathy*)

>> *Anemia* (low red blood cell count)

>> Low platelet count

Given the many risks associated with drinking, especially its effect on high blood pressure, reducing your consumption of alcohol — or quitting altogether — is key.

If you think you might have a drinking problem, or you're having trouble cutting back on or quitting alcohol, check out *Addiction & Recovery For Dummies*, 2nd Edition, by Paul Ritvo (published by Wiley).

Cutting Back on Caffeine

Caffeine is a chemical compound in the leaves, seeds, and fruits of more than 63 plant species, but it most commonly comes from coffee and cocoa beans, cola nuts, and tea leaves. Coffee isn't the only source of caffeine — a can of cola contains 45 mg of caffeine, green tea has 30 mg, and an ounce of chocolate has 20 mg.

Caffeine produces an increase in blood pressure for about three hours after you consume it. If you consume more than 200 mg of caffeine per day, systolic blood pressure rises by an average of 8 mmHg and diastolic blood pressure rises by an average of approximately 5 mmHg.

A study of more than 250,000 women found that those who drank the most caffeine-containing drinks (including coffee and sodas) tended to have the highest blood pressure.

In a study involving more than 700 patients, people who had already been diagnosed with high blood pressure and consumed more than three cups of coffee a day were found to be at increased risk of developing *resistant* (difficult to control) high blood pressure. The take-home point regarding caffeine is that if you've been diagnosed with high blood pressure, you may be more sensitive to the blood-pressure-raising effects of caffeine. This blood pressure rise is then sustained. This effect is particularly true for older people.

REMEMBER

A 5 mm Hg rise in blood pressure may sound trivial, but it results in a 21 percent increase in the incidence of heart disease (see Chapter 5) and a 34 percent increase in the incidence of stroke (see Chapter 7). In addition, when taken with alcohol or tobacco, which is so often the case, the combination greatly increases the blood-pressure-raising effect.

TIP

Don't have a cup of coffee before you go to have your blood pressure measured or before a medical office visit. The temporary elevation in blood pressure may convince your health-care provider that you have high blood pressure.

Knowing how much is too much

The daily recommended maximum amount of caffeine is 300 mg, and an ordinary cup of coffee (5 ounces) has 100 mg of caffeine. However:

>> An 8-ounce cup of coffee at a nice cafe or fancy coffee shop contains 250 mg of caffeine, more than double the amount of that ordinary cup.

>> A 12-ounce cup of coffee from the same shop has 375 mg of caffeine, nearly four times that ordinary cup.

>> A 16-ounce cup of coffee packs 550 mg of caffeine, more than five times the punch.

You can see where a few cups of coffee can quickly add up to much more than the daily recommended maximum.

Considering caffeine's health consequences

Caffeine is a mildly addictive drug. When you stop drinking it, you have withdrawal symptoms, such as:

>> Feelings of sleepiness

>> Feelings of being overtired

>> Severe headache

But caffeine also has a number of potential medical consequences when a person consumes it in large doses (over 300 mg daily) over a period of years:

>> **Osteoporosis (thinning of the bone):** As a result of the urine-promoting effect of caffeine, the calcium that a body needs to build strong bones passes quickly into the urine. If you're a regular caffeine drinker, make sure to get extra calcium from other sources like dairy products or calcium pills.

>> **Infertility, birth defects, and miscarriages.**

>> **Heartburn and even ulcers due to increased stomach acid production.**

>> **Increased risk of heart disease when coffee is unfiltered.**

>> **Increased premenstrual pain and formation of breast lumps (but these findings are controversial).**

>> **Poor sleep quality and difficulty falling asleep.**

REMEMBER

Caffeine can keep you awake, but it does *not* improve your performance of complex tasks.

Recognizing the gains in giving up caffeine

When you give up caffeine, you reduce your chances of developing any of the conditions in the preceding section, you eliminate an unnecessary drug from your body, *and* you help keep your blood pressure under control. If you're a woman, you may greatly enhance your chances of becoming pregnant and having a healthy pregnancy and delivery.

Avoiding the beans, chocolate, energy drinks, and soda

If you consume no more than two cups of coffee daily, you should have no symptoms if you switch to decaffeinated drinks and avoid other sources of caffeine like chocolate. If you have a history of high blood pressure, be very careful when consuming energy drinks that can have a high amount of caffeine. Talk with your health-care provider if you fall into this category.

If you consume a lot more caffeine daily, the process of quitting may be more difficult. Here are some suggestions:

>> **Try to determine how much caffeine you're taking in each day.** Check all foods and medications to make sure you're not missing an unexpected source.

>> **Reduce your intake and see how you feel as you withdraw.**

>> **Gradually reduce your daily caffeine by 50 mg or so until you're free of it.**

>> **Use exercise to give you the energy you believe was coming from caffeine.** If you're able to take a walk during lunch, that may help reset you for the rest of the afternoon so you don't need the caffeine.

>> **Avoid the other habits such as smoking that go with drinking coffee.**

>> **Ask the people you live and eat with to help you by reducing their caffeine intake.** The improvement they feel will make them grateful.

IN THIS CHAPTER

» Noting the value of exercise

» Getting started

» Knowing your limits and seeing your health-care provider

» Exercising for weight loss and strength

» Lowering your blood pressure with alternative measures

Chapter **12**

Lowering Blood Pressure with Exercise

B lood pressure medication is an important treatment for high blood pressure, but exercise is just as important if not more so. When I'm working with a patient who has high blood pressure, in addition to writing a prescription for medication, I also write a prescription for beginning an exercise program.

The benefits of a regular exercise program can't be denied. If you have high blood pressure, exercise can lower it. If you don't have high blood pressure, exercise can prevent it. Plus, exercise can help you maintain a healthy weight, decrease your waist circumference (an important aspect of metabolic syndrome, which can lead to the development of diabetes), and also improve your energy levels!

This chapter fills you in on all the benefits of exercise and physical activity.

Recognizing the Benefits of Exercise

Exercise strengthens all the muscles involved in your body's movement. If you walk or jog, you strengthen your leg muscles. If you lift weights, you strengthen your arm muscles. Whatever the exercise, your heart — which is also a muscle — becomes stronger. At the same time, your body opens up your arteries to allow for more flow of nutrients into the tissues. The combination of a stronger, more efficient heart and more open blood vessels leads to lower blood pressure.

Lowering your blood pressure is a good enough reason to make exercise an important part of your lifestyle, but here are some more reasons for beginning an exercise program. Exercise helps to:

» Improve your memory

» Reduce your risk of cancer

» Lower your blood sugar, helping to protect against developing diabetes

» Increase your energy level

» Improve your mood

» Help you sleep better and longer (which is associated with lower blood pressure and improved quality of life)

» Strengthen your bones

» Improve your cholesterol levels (by lowering "bad" cholesterol and raising "good" cholesterol)

TIP

You may have heard that "sitting is the new smoking." Health-care professionals use this phrase to remind people of the dangers of a sedentary lifestyle. If you're sitting six to eight hours a day, get up and walk around at least once an hour. You may be thinking to yourself, "But I exercise several times a week." Above and beyond any exercise program you may be doing, you still need to get up and walk around at least once an hour.

Preparing to Begin an Exercise Program

Before beginning an exercise program, especially if you're older or more sedentary, preparation is important. Take these important steps before you begin an exercise program:

1. **Go for a checkup with your doctor to make sure your body can handle an exercise program.**

2. **Choose the exercises that you plan to make part of your program.**

3. **Get the right equipment.**

Getting a checkup

Before beginning an exercise program, you need to know where you stand health-wise. If you haven't been exercising on a regular basis, talk with your health-care provider to determine the right level of exercise to begin with. Talk about past and current medical problems, review any medications and supplements you take, get an assessment of your physical capabilities, and let them know which exercises you have in mind. Your health-care provider is your ally in developing an exercise program!

If you have heart disease, your health-care provider may recommend further cardiac testing, including an electrocardiogram (ECG) or a stress test, to assess the response of your heart to fairly vigorous exercise. If you get through a stress test without developing symptoms such as chest pain, severe shortness of breath, or changes in your ECG, you're likely in decent enough physical condition to begin an exercise program.

REMEMBER

No matter what type of exercise program you choose, please note the following:

>> **Start slowly and build up over time.** You don't need to rush to get to a certain level of exercise by a certain date. Take it one day at a time, especially if you haven't exercised on a regular basis before. Rome wasn't built in a day, and it will take time to improve your overall health. Allow yourself the time to gradually work your way along until you achieve your goal.

>> **Exercise on a regular basis can have a more sustained effect on blood pressure.** Regular exercise several times a week has a more profound effect on blood pressure than exercising only one or two days a week.

WARNING

If you develop any dizziness or lightheadedness during or after exercise, check your blood pressure and talk with your doctor. You may need to adjust the time you're taking your blood pressure medications in relation to when you exercise.

REMEMBER

As you get more fit and/or lose weight, your blood pressure will likely improve and your blood pressure medication requirements may need to be reduced.

Personalizing your exercise program

For maximum effect, most exercise programs combine two types of exercise:

» **Aerobic:** *Aerobic* means "with oxygen." During aerobic exercise, the body uses oxygen to help provide energy. Aerobic activity can be sustained for more than a few minutes, and it involves major groups of muscles (particularly the legs, but also the arms). Activities such as walking, running, cycling, tennis, basketball, and so forth make your heart pump faster during the exercise.

» **Anaerobic:** *Anaerobic* means "without oxygen." Anaerobic exercises are very intense, so they can't be sustained for very long. Anaerobic exercises depend on sources of energy that are already available (like glucose in your muscle). These include high-intensity exercises. Examples are lifting heavy weights and doing the 100-yard dash.

If you're wondering which category strength training falls into, here's the answer: Both! Strength training can have an aerobic component (if you use a lower weight and do more repetitions) or an anaerobic component (if you use heavy weight and do fewer repetitions).

REMEMBER

Engaging in a regular aerobic exercise program can, over time, lower your systolic blood pressure (the top number of the blood pressure) up to 5 to 7 points and help you to decrease the amount of blood pressure medications you're taking. An exercise program that combines the different kinds of exercise helps to give you the best of both worlds — lower blood pressure and stronger muscles.

EXERCISING AT THE RIGHT INTENSITY LEVEL

There are many different levels of intensity when it comes to exercise. One way to determine the intensity level of your exercise is the *perceived exertion scale*, which can help you figure out if the exercise you're doing is actually improving your fitness.

How do you rate the degree of exertion and intensity? You rate the degree of your exertion while performing a certain activity using one of the following categories:

• **Very light:** This is like walking slowly for several minutes.

• **Fairly light:** At this level, you're breathing harder, but you can continue.

- **Somewhat difficult:** The exercise is getting a little difficult, but it still feels okay to continue.

- **Difficult:** You're starting to have trouble breathing; speaking is difficult.

- **Very difficult:** The exercise is difficult to continue, so you have to push yourself; you're very tired and you're having trouble talking comfortably.

- **Extremely difficult:** This is the most difficult exercise you've ever tried.

As your fitness level increases, your ratings of various exercises will change, too. What was once *very difficult* may become *fairly light.*

If you're contemplating adding a high-intensity exercise component to your routine, talk with your doctor to make sure it's safe for you to do. They may recommend a stress test to better determine your ability to handle high-intensity exercise, especially if you have a heart condition.

Mixing in higher-intensity exercise does have benefits, including improving fitness, strength, and endurance. It also increases your risk of injury, depending on the exercise and its intensity. All the more reason to talk with your health-care provider before embarking on an exercise program.

Remember: You don't have to do high-intensity exercise to lower your blood pressure. Begin at the light to fairly light stage and see how you feel. Talk with your doctor about increasing your exercise intensity with the goal of gradually increasing it.

Walking for exercise

Walking is an exercise that almost everyone can perform. You don't have to belong to a special club or organization, and, unless you live in an area that has snow a good portion of the year, you can walk outside most any day — even in the rain. You can walk alone or walk with others, but walking with a friend not only makes the activity more pleasant but also allows you to encourage each other to stay committed.

Table 12-1 outlines one walking program that starts slowly; most people can complete Level 1 without a great deal of difficulty. (If you need to, just begin slowly and only go ½ mile. The key is regular, purposeful movement each and every day.) After you've completed one level, you're ready to move to the next level.

TIP

How do you know where to start? The best way is to walk a mile at your normal walking pace and record how long it takes. That's your starting point.

Table 12-1 breaks the walking program into 15 levels so you can work your way up to a desired level of fitness to lower your blood pressure. Take your time and enjoy the journey. The journey of a thousand miles does indeed begin with a single step.

TABLE 12-1

Suggested Walking Program to Lower Blood Pressure

Level	Distance (in Miles)	Time (in Minutes)
1	1	30
2	1	28
3	1	26
4	1	24
5	1	22
6	1	20
7	1½	32
8	1½	31
9	1½	30
10	1½	29
11	1½	28
12	1½	27
13	1½	26
14	1½	25
15	1½	24

Thirty minutes a day is a recommended length of exercise. When you reach Level 15, you want to maintain this ideally for the rest of your life. It will make a significant difference in your blood pressure, as well as improve other aspects of your health. Thirty minutes a day to make high blood pressure go away!

TIP

An alternative to the 15-level program is walking 10,000 steps a day. One way to record your steps is to use a *pedometer,* a device that counts your steps. You can buy pedometers that you clip on your waistband,you're your smartphone or smart watches may already be tracking your steps for you. Keep track of your daily steps for a week to get your average daily steps. Then try to increase your steps by 500 steps per day and do that for a week before increasing by 500 steps again. When you've gone seven days at this new level, go for another 500. Keep increasing until you've reached 10,000 steps a day.

Choosing other aerobic activities

Walking is great exercise and certainly one of the easiest to do, but there are many different options out there. The idea of personalizing an exercise program is to pick one you *enjoy* doing. If you prefer other types of aerobically effective activities, go for it! Just make sure you can physically do a certain exercise *and* stick with it. Table 12-2 lists some of those options, as well as the amount of calories burned with each type of activity.

In addition, consider biking, cricket, dancing, handball, judo, karate, pickleball, racquetball, rowing, rugby, soccer, squash, swimming, and tennis (singles is better than doubles because you have to run around more). What you do doesn't really matter. You just need to do *something*.

Using the right equipment

Depending on the exercise you choose to participate in, be sure to get the right equipment. If you plan to engage in an exercise such as walking and/or jogging for example, having the proper footwear is important. Footwear can be a little pricey, but when you remember the benefits to your feet, knees, and hips, you'll see that they're well worth the price.

TIP

Try to find a store where the staff is knowledgeable about shoe needs, perhaps one that caters to runners and walkers.

Make sure you have the right exercise clothing. Dressing in layers is a good idea because you can remove clothing as needed. Some sports clothes are better than others because they allow your perspiration to pass through and evaporate rather than sticking to your body. This process cools you off and helps you to feel less wet as you exercise. (Cotton absorbs sweat and holds it against your skin, which isn't ideal.) For cooler weather, choose an outer layer that repels wind and rain but allows sweat to pass through.

If you're into biking, make sure you have the right bike suitable for the right terrain. Bikes that are good for street biking are very different from mountain bikes. Even the tires are different. If you want to limit yourself to an indoor stationary cycle, make sure the quality is good. Plenty of resources such as *Consumer Reports* magazine are available to guide your decision. You can also find help on the internet. Two excellent resources are Road Bike Review (www.roadbikereview.com) and Mountain Bike Review (www.mtbr.com).

Exercising to Lose Weight

Exercise can help you lose weight, but you need to exercise at least 90 minutes six days a week. To maintain a weight loss, you need to do 60 minutes daily. To improve your physical conditioning and have an effect on your blood pressure, you need at least 30 minutes a day.

TIP

The exercise doesn't need to be continuous. Three ten-minute sessions are as good as 30 uninterrupted minutes.

REMEMBER

A kilocalorie (or calorie for short) is the amount of energy needed to raise the temperature of a kilogram of water 1 degree centigrade. One pound of fat contains 3,500 calories. So, to lose a pound of fat, you must use (burn, exercise, whatever) at least 3,500 calories more than you eat. For example, if you eat 2,000 calories a day to maintain your weight, you can lose 1 pound in seven days by using 500 calories more each day than usual ($500 \times 7 = 3,500$). Doing only 250 calories of extra exercise takes 14 days to lose the same pound. Walking an hour each day burns 4 calories per minute, 240 calories in all.

Table 12-2 shows the number of calories that you burn doing several different kinds of exercise for 30, 45, or 60 minutes.

TABLE 12-2 **Calories Burned Doing Various Exercises**

Activity	30 Minutes	45 Minutes	60 Minutes
Tennis (doubles)	85	128	170
Walking a 20-minute mile on a flat surface	120	180	240
Water aerobics	140	210	280
Walking a 15-minute mile on a flat surface	146	219	292
Walking a 20-minute mile uphill	162	243	324
Golf (carrying your bag)	174	261	348
Walking a 15-minute mile uphill	206	309	412
Swimming	250	375	500
Basketball	282	423	564
Bicycling 12 miles per hour	283	425	566
Cross-country skiing	291	438	583
Aerobic dance	342	513	684
Running a 10-minute mile	365	549	732

Exercising to Gain Strength

A complete exercise program includes aerobic exercise to lower your blood pressure and resistance training to strengthen your muscles. Strengthening your muscles allows you to do more aerobic exercise. It also improves your balance. Resistance training complements aerobic exercise by improving muscle strength, endurance, and flexibility. This is so important, especially as you get older. Unless your doctor says otherwise, your personalized exercise program should include some resistance training a few times a week. Many people use very light free weights or exercise bands. You can even lift cans of soup (just check the sodium content of the soup before consuming the contents within!).

TIP

Talk with your doctor before beginning any type of strength training. If you have prior orthopedic or joint-related injuries or a medical condition involving the muscle or joints, there may be certain exercises that you shouldn't do (as well as exercises that you *should* do). If your health-care provider gives you the green light to embark on an exercise program, talk to a personal trainer if you have questions. Many hospitals and health networks have gyms with exercise personnel in them to help you start an exercise program safely. They can perform additional personalized testing to get a real sense of your physical capabilities and limitations and help you design a safe personal exercise program.

WARNING

If you have high blood pressure, use lighter weights that allow you to do many repetitions of an exercise instead of a few extreme lifts with very heavy weights. Extreme lifting may suddenly raise your blood pressure to unacceptable levels. You don't want to start any exercise program lifting heavy weights, especially if you haven't lifted before and especially if you have high blood pressure.

Lowering Your Blood Pressure with Complementary Therapies

Although aerobic exercise is extremely helpful for lowering blood pressure, other disciplines can help accomplish this goal as well. When combined with exercise, the results can be significant.

TIP

Yoga, meditation, hypnosis, and biofeedback are common therapies for treating high blood pressure, but they aren't the only options. Check out the National Center for Complementaty and Integrative Health (www.nccih.nih.gov/health/hypertension-high-blood-pressure) for other options regarding alternative and complementary medicine.

Yoga

Yoga is a series of postures and breathing exercises developed in India over 5,000 years ago as a way to achieve *union* (or *yoga*) with the divine consciousness. Today, people often practice yoga as a way of improving their health and well-being. Yoga attempts to unite your body and your mind so your mind can function better in a healthier body. Numerous studies have shown that yoga can lower blood pressure; this effect persists as long as the practice continues, and it often disappears if the person stops practicing yoga.

Over its 5,000-year existence, yoga has evolved in many directions as teachers have developed their different philosophies. As a result, yoga has eight main branches. *Hatha yoga,* the most popular branch, emphasizes physical fitness more than the others do.

TIP

An excellent source of information about all aspects of yoga is *Yoga For Dummies* by Brenda Feuerstein and Larry Payne (Wiley). I highly recommend it. The internet also offers many excellent yoga websites. Three of the many excellent sites available include the following:

>> **Yoga with Adriene:** Yoga instructor Adriene Mishler offers hundreds of yoga videos on her YouTube channel (www.youtube.com/@yogawithadriene). If you're new to yoga, check out one of her videos for beginners, like this one: https://youtu.be/j7rKKpwdXNE.

>> **Yoga Basics:** This website can answer many of your questions about yoga. Check it out at www.yogabasics.com.

>> *Yoga Journal: Yoga Journal* has numerous articles concerning the world of yoga. Find it at www.yogajournal.com.

Meditation

Meditation involves concentrating on an object, a sound, a word, or the breath in order to diminish random thoughts and improve focus. The result is a calmer, more peaceful mind. Meditation doesn't involve specific body postures like yoga does, but some aspects of yoga involve meditation, particularly the awareness of the breath.

DEEP BREATHING

One important exercise that you can do every day to not only help you relax but also lower your blood pressure is deep breathing. Deep breathing is not only a good way to help reduce the effect of "white-coat hypertension" (see Chapter 2), but also delay or even inhibit the fight-or-flight response that can increases blood pressure during a stressful event.

Build deep breathing into your routine a couple of times a day if possible. All you have to do is sit down, close your eyes, inhale deeply for a count of four, hold your breath for a count of four, and then exhale slowly for a count of four. Repeat this four times in one sitting. The more you do this throughout your day, the better you become at it and the more natural it seems. Deep breathing is also a way to calm yourself during a stressful event.

Meditation may be the best studied of the various forms of relaxation. Articles in the *American Journal of Hypertension* (May 2005) and the *American Journal of Cardiology* (January 2005) compare meditation with other forms of relaxation and find that the effect of meditation is significant in lowering blood pressure, much better than muscle relaxation and mental relaxation. Many clinical studies have shown that meditation can lower blood pressure and keep it reduced as long as the practice is continued.

TIP

Just like yoga, meditation has gone in different directions over the years. The most popular form is transcendental meditation. You can find out much more about this technique by reading *Meditation For Dummies* by Stephan Bodian (Wiley). Examples of some common meditation apps that you can download and use include Headspace (www.headspace.com) and Calm (www.calm.com).

Biofeedback

Biofeedback is a technique developed in the late 1960s in which you train yourself to alter an *involuntary function* (like heart rate, body temperature, or blood pressure) with the aid of a *biofeedback machine.* Biofeedback machines detect a person's internal bodily functions so the functions can be altered.

For example, one biofeedback machine picks up electrical signals from muscles and translates them into a flashing light. In order to reduce the tension in their muscles, the person using the machine first figures out how to slow down the flashes of light. After a while, they no longer need the machine to relax; they simply use the methods they discovered with the machine.

TIP

Various kinds of equipment are available for biofeedback, and numerous websites can help you find them, including the following:

>> **The Association for Applied Psychophysiology and Biofeedback** (`https://aapb.org`): This website has answers to common questions, as well as a list of practitioners, a bookstore, and links to more information.

>> **Mayo Clinic Biofeedback Overview** (`www.mayoclinic.org/tests-procedures/biofeedback/about/pac-20384664`): The Mayo Clinic website is an online source for information about a variety of health-related subjects, including biofeedback.

Chapter **13**

Taking Medications to Lower Your Blood Pressure

Nutrition and exercise are the first steps in preventing and treating high blood pressure. But often — especially if you already have high blood pressure — they aren't enough on their own, and you'll need to take a prescription medication in order to get your blood pressure under control.

This chapter reviews the many different medications your doctor may prescribe. The goal of this chapter is to give you all the information you need about these medications so, when you see your doctor, you can be your own advocate and have an informed discussion about the options.

REMEMBER

If you're taking medication to help lower your blood pressure, diet and exercise are still important — you aren't let off the hook on those fronts! Often, when your diet and exercise routines are in order, you won't have to take as much medication.

REMEMBER

Talking with your doctor is key, especially when starting a new medication. If a blood pressure medication isn't working for you — either because it's not effective or because you're experiencing some nasty side effects from it — reach out to your doctor. Don't stop taking the medication unless your doctor tells you to. With some medications, if you stop them suddenly, it can cause a dangerous spike in blood pressure.

TIP

While you're taking medication for high blood pressure, check your blood pressure at home both sitting and standing, at least once a day and record the measurements. Dizziness upon standing is a common symptom of many if not all the medications in this chapter. It can also be a sign of dehydration (if you're on diuretics) or a blood pressure that may be too low (if you're on other blood pressure medications). This information will be important for your doctor so they can fine-tune your medication regimen.

Examining Classes of Blood Pressure Medications

Medications that lower blood pressure are divided into several classes: diuretics, angiotensin-converting enzyme (ACE) inhibitors, angiotensin II receptor blockers (ARBs), calcium channel blockers (CCBs), medications that act on the nervous system, and vasodilators. Each class works differently.

TIP

Some side effects can be attributed to an entire medication class (for example, cough can be a significant side effect of any medication among ACE inhibitors). Other side effects differ even among medications in the same class.

The medications in this chapter are categorized according to the way that they lower blood pressure. The medications in this chapter are referred to by their generic names (that is, their official chemical designations), as well as their brand names.

REMEMBER

I list the brand names in parentheses after the generic names throughout the chapter. However, because you probably know a drug by its brand name, you can find information on it faster by checking out the alphabetical listing of brand names with their generic names at the end of this chapter.

Diuretics: Medications that reduce fluid buildup

Diuretics, also known as "water pills," lower blood pressure through the elimination of sodium and water through the kidneys into the urine. There are different types of diuretics, and they're used by doctors for different reasons. Here are the types of diuretics:

>> **Thiazide and thiazide-like diuretics:** Thiazide and thiazide-like diuretics are first-line agents for the treatment of blood pressure. They're not the most effective drugs for ridding the body of excess salt and water, but they *are* the most effective for lowering blood pressure.

>> **Loop diuretics:** Loop diuretics are excellent in helping the kidneys to get rid of excess salt and water. They're used for people who have congestive heart failure or other conditions (including chronic kidney disease), to prevent the buildup of excess swelling called *edema*. Although loop diuretics are great for getting rid of excess fluid, they aren't as good as thiazide diuretics for blood pressure control.

>> **Potassium-sparing diuretics:** Potassium-sparing diuretics are good for the treatment of blood pressure, and they have other beneficial effects, too. They aren't first-line agents for blood pressure, but they're often used when other medications aren't effective. They're also used to help maintain normal potassium levels in the body when used with other medications (other diuretics cause potassium loss).

>> **Aldosterone-antagonist group:** This is a special group of potassium-sparing diuretics that block the action of *aldosterone,* a natural blood pressure hormone that causes salt and water retention.

Thiazide and thiazide-like diuretics

Thiazide diuretics, a first-line agent for the treatment of high blood pressure, have been prescribed for more than 30 years and have the following positive characteristics:

>> You only need to take them once a day.

>> They're very inexpensive.

>> They're effective in lower doses, which helps reduce the potential for side effects.

>> They're well tolerated.

>> They're very effective in salt-sensitive high blood pressure.

>> If you're taking another class of blood pressure medications and your doctor adds a thiazide diuretic, it can increase the blood-pressure-lowering effects of the other medication, and the two medications together can really improve your blood pressure.

>> Because they can lower calcium levels in the urine, they're used in the treatment of kidney stones. So, if you have high blood pressure and kidney stones, you get a double benefit from them.

Common side effects of thiazide diuretics include the following:

>> They cause increased urination at night, which can cause you to get less sleep. This side effect can be minimized by taking the medication earlier in the day.

>> The reduction in urinary calcium excretion may raise your blood levels of calcium. Higher-than-normal levels of calcium can cause side effects. Your doctor will check your bloodwork after starting this medication to make sure your electrolytes are okay.

>> They aren't recommended during pregnancy and while breastfeeding.

>> They can cause electrolyte abnormalities, including low potassium levels, low sodium levels, and higher glucose levels, as well as higher calcium levels (as noted earlier). Very low potassium levels can cause symptoms such as diffuse weakness, muscle cramping and pains, nausea, and vomiting. Signs and symptoms of very low sodium levels can include weakness, confusion, falls, dizziness, nausea, and vomiting; the symptoms are more severe the lower the sodium levels are. If you experience any of these side effects, tell your doctor right away.

>> They can increase uric acid levels in the blood. If you have a history of gout, you may be at increased risk of developing this condition.

>> In some men, they can cause erectile dysfunction, especially in higher doses.

>> Thiazide diuretics are sulfa-related, so if you have an allergy to sulfa medications (such as the antibiotic trimethoprim-sulfamethoxizale [brand name: Bactrim]), you may not be able to take thiazide diuretics.

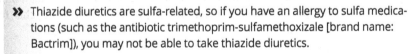

Anti-inflammatory drugs, like ibuprofen and naproxen, cause salt and water retention. If you're taking thiazide diuretics at the same time, the blood-pressure–lowering effects of these medications can be reduced by anti-inflammatory medications. If you have high blood pressure and are on medications like ibuprofen or naproxen, let your doctor know.

The following sections review some of the more commonly prescribed medications in this class.

HYDROCHLOROTHIAZIDE

Of all the thiazide diuretics, hydrochlorothiazide (brand names: HydroDIURIL, Hydrochlorothiazide Capsules, Hydrochlorothiazide Oral Solution, and Hydrochlorothiazide Tablets) is probably prescribed the most often. It's relatively inexpensive, and it's commonly taken once a day. Hydrochlorothiazide has proven its value over many years and is effective in small doses. It's less effective for high blood pressure in people who have chronic kidney disease with kidney function of 35 percent or less; for this reason, it's prescribed with caution in people with chronic kidney disease.

This medication can be prescribed as low as 12.5 mg a day with most health care practitioners prescribing at 25 mg daily.

CHLORTHALIDONE

Chlorthalidone (brand names: Thalitone, Chlorthalidone Tablets) differs chemically from hydrochlorothiazide, and its effects tend to last longer, but its blood-pressure-lowering activity is about the same. The precautions associated with hydrochlorothiazide also pertain to chlorthalidone, which comes in 15-, 25-, 50- and 100-milligram tablets. Taking half of the smallest tablet may be enough to control blood pressure. It's taken once daily.

INDAPAMIDE

Indapamide (brand name: Indapamide Tablets) is more like chlorthalidone than hydrochlorothiazide in its structure, but it has 20 times the potency of hydrochlorothiazide. Because it doesn't raise serum cholesterol, indapamide has an advantage over hydrochlorothiazide.

Indapamide is available at a dose of 1.5 or 2.5 mg with the usual once- or twice-daily treatment. However, a sustained-release preparation contains 1.5 mg that lasts throughout a 24-hour period with less effect on the potassium than the higher dosage. The 1.5-milligram dosage is just as effective as 2 and 2.5 mg.

METOLAZONE

Metolazone (brand names: Mykrox, Zaroxolyn, Metolazone Tablets) is structurally different from hydrochlorothiazide but acts in much the same way. It's more potent than hydrochlorothiazide.

Mykrox has an advantage over Zaroxolyn and other diuretics because of its rapid absorption and earlier activity. Although Zaroxolyn is the same drug as Mykrox, Zaroxolyn is absorbed more slowly and isn't interchangeable with Mykrox. Mykrox comes in 0.5-milligram tablets. Zaroxolyn comes in 2.5-, 5-, and 10-milligram dosages taken once a day. The precautions for both meds are the same as for hydrochlorothiazide.

Loop diuretics

Loop diuretics are more effective than the thiazide diuretics for ridding the body of salt and water, but they aren't as good at lowering blood pressure. They're used in the treatment of conditions that can cause fluid to build up, such as congestive heart failure and advanced kidney disease.

Other issues associated with loop diuretics include the following:

>> Some people can develop hearing loss and/or a ringing in the ears when taking them. This is not a common side effect, but when it occurs, the hearing loss and/or ringing in the ears can persist despite stopping the medications. If you're taking a loop diuretic, be aware of other medications that can affect your hearing, such as aspirin and some antibiotics — loop diuretics may cause even more damage. Talk with your doctor or pharmacist if you have any questions about medications that you're taking and possible interactions or side effects.

>> Your doctor should check your blood level of sodium, potassium, calcium, and magnesium frequently during your first few months on loop diuretics.

>> They can increase uric acid levels in the blood. If you have a history of gout, you may be at increased risk of developing this condition.

>> In people who are hypersensitive to several sulfa-containing antibiotics and sulfonamides, reactions can occur.

>> Some other medications interact with loop diuretics. These include the following:

- Anti-inflammatory drugs like ibuprofen and naproxen. Because anti-inflammatory drugs cause salt and water retention, they blunt the blood-pressure-lowering effects of loop diuretics.

- Warfarin (brand name: Coumadin). There is an important interaction between one of the loop diuretics (Torsemide) and Warfarin (a blood thinner) that can increase the Warfarin levels and bleeding risk. This is not seen with other loop diuretics.

Loop diuretics are not commonly recommended during pregnancy. In pregnant women, they're only used when really, really necessary. Talk with your doctor before taking this class of medications when you're pregnant.

If you're on any loop diuretic, weigh yourself every day at the same time of day and record your weight. If you notice your weight increasing by more than 2 pounds a day for two days (or 4 to 5 pounds over two days), call your doctor and see if your medication needs to be adjusted.

Although loop diuretics can have an effect on blood pressure (especially if there is swelling present), thiazide and thiazide-like diuretics are better for high blood pressure.

The following sections take a brief look at commonly prescribed loop diuretics.

FUROSEMIDE

Furosemide (brand names: Lasix, Furosemide Tablets, Furosemide Oral Solution) is the most commonly used loop diuretic. It eliminates excess salt and water from the body — in fact, it can cause salt loss and dehydration. Other important considerations when it comes to furosemide include the following:

>> If you're taking lithium, furosemide can cause dehydration. Your kidney function and electrolytes will need to be monitored if you're on lithium and a loop diuretic like furosemide.

>> Sucralfate, a drug used for the treatment of stomach ulcers, may decrease the effect of furosemide. Wait two hours after taking sucralfate before taking furosemide.

Furosemide comes in 20-, 40-, and 80-milligram tablets. Many patients are prescribed the lowest dose at first. It usually begins to work in about one to two hours, with peak effect in six hours. You may be told to take it from once a day up to even three or four times a day, but once or twice a day is most common.

ETHACRYNIC ACID

Ethacrynic acid (brand name: Edecrin Tablets) is similar in structure to furosemide but is slightly less potent. It shares the problems of this powerful group of diuretics and should probably not be used during pregnancy or breastfeeding.

Ethacrynic acid comes in 25- and 50-milligram tablets taken one to three times a day as needed. For high blood pressure, 25 mg should be taken after a meal. It usually starts to work within 30 minutes and lasts for about eight hours.

This is the one loop diuretic that is not sulfa related. If you have a sulfa allergy and need a diuretic for fluid management, your doctor may suggest this medication for you.

TORSEMIDE

Torsemide (brand name: Demadex) has three times the potency of furosemide and is thought to be the best absorbed of all the loop diuretics. The liver does most of the metabolizing of this drug, so torsemide is particularly dangerous if you have severe liver disease.

Torsemide is available as 5-, 10-, 20-, and 100-milligram tablets taken once a day initially. You can take it at any time of day (no need to consider meal times); it usually begins to work in an hour and lasts about 12 hours.

This medication interacts with Warfarin and can increase the Warfarin levels and subsequent bleeding risk.

BUMETANIDE

Bumetanide (brand names: Bumex, Bumetanide Tablets) is similar in structure and side effects to furosemide but is 40 times more potent. It's better absorbed than furosemide in its oral form.

Bumetanide is available as 0.5-, 1-, and 2-milligram tablets. It usually begins to work in 30 to 60 minutes and lasts about six hours. Patients usually take it once a day in the morning, but if a single dose doesn't work long enough, your doctor may prescribe a second dose later in the day (before 6 p.m. to avoid waking up to having to go to the bathroom overnight).

Potassium-sparing diuretics

Potassium-sparing diuretics are effective at controlling blood pressure but are not first-line agents for blood control. (Aldosterone antagonist diuretics are potassium-sparing diuretics, but they're so unique that I discuss them separately.) Often the two potassium diuretics in this section, amiloride and triamterene, are combined with a thiazide diuretic — the thiazide diuretics can cause potassium loss, but the potassium-sparing diuretics help to counter this effect.

Their ability to conserve potassium can also lead to an abnormal elevation of the blood-potassium level, so they should never be used if your potassium level is already high. If you start taking a medication in this class, your doctor should check your bloodwork before and after starting it to get a baseline potassium level and kidney function. If you have kidney disease, your doctor is less likely to prescribe medications in this class.

AMILORIDE

Amiloride (brand name: Midamor Tablets, Amiloride HCl Tablets) has been around for a while. It's usually only prescribed when many other medications haven't worked. It also can be used to help in the treatment of low magnesium levels.

WARNING

Amiloride can cause excessive potassium retention, so your doctor will want to monitor your blood potassium levels. If you have kidney disease and/or diabetes, the risk of high potassium levels can be greater, so your doctor will want to keep an eye on that.

This drug comes in a 5-milligram tablets. It starts to act in 2 hours and continues its activity for 24 hours.

TRIAMTERENE

Triamterene (brand name: Dyrenium) differs in structure from amiloride and has only one-tenth of amiloride's potency. It accomplishes the same task of conserving potassium in people who are taking a diuretic that causes potassium loss. This medication is more commonly prescribed as part of a combination medication with hydrochlorothiazide called Dyazide. Like Amiloride, this is an older medication, and it's less commonly prescribed.

WARNING

Triamterene can cause kidney stones in some people. If you have a history of kidney stones, talk with your doctor before taking this medication. The same warnings regarding high potassium levels that apply to amiloride also apply to triamterene.

Triamterene comes as 50- and 100-milligram tablets, usually starts to act in two to four hours, and lasts up to nine hours. As a result, people usually need to take it twice a day, which is a disadvantage. It's often taken after meals to avoid stomach upset.

Aldosterone-antagonist diuretics

Aldosterone-antagonist diuretics do not directly cause loss of salt and potassium in the urine. Instead, they block the action of the steroid hormone aldosterone (see Chapter 4), which causes salt and water retention. They also conserve potassium, so these are also potassium-sparing medications.

If your potassium level is already elevated or you're taking a drug that tends to raise potassium, your doctor will want to watch your potassium levels closely.

All the risks associated with high potassium levels for the potassium-sparing diuretics (see the previous section) apply to aldosterone-antagonist diuretics.

Because these medications antagonize the actions of aldosterone (see Chapter 4), they have cardiac and kidney protective effects.

SPIRONOLACTONE

Spironolactone (brand name: Aldactone) has a number of possible side effects you should be aware of:

>> Breast enlargement in men and women

>> Nipple tenderness

>> Erectile dysfunction

>> Decreased interest in sex

>> Increased hairiness

>> Deepening of the voice

>> Menstrual irregularities

>> Sleepiness

>> Confusion

>> Headaches

>> Irritation and bleeding in the stomach

The drug comes in 25-, 50-, and 100-milligram tablets, usually starts to act only after one to two days, and continues to increase salt and urine output for two to three days. For high blood pressure, patients usually take 50 mg once a day, along with a diuretic that causes potassium loss. Your doctor may be willing to reduce the dose to 25 mg with a good result.

EPLERENONE

Eplerenone (brand name: Inspra) is a newer aldosterone antagonist with far fewer side effects than spironolactone (eplerenone doesn't cause breast enlargement or sexual side effects). It comes in 25- and 50-milligram tablets. The dose starts at 50 mg and is given once or twice a day as needed. The potassium level is monitored on a weekly basis.

Other first-line medications

In addition to the thiazide diuretics, ACE inhibitors, ARBs, and CCBs are considered first-line agents for the treatment of high blood pressure. I go into detail on all of these in this section.

DIURETIC COMBINATIONS

Because of the thiazide diuretics' tendency to cause potassium loss, a number of medication combinations are available:

- **Amiloride Hydrochloride and Hydrochlorothiazide Tablets:** 5 mg of amiloride and 50 mg of hydrochlorothiazide

- **Dyazide:** 37.5 mg of triamterene and 25 mg of hydrochlorothiazide

- **Maxide:** 75 mg of triamterene and 50 mg of hydrochlorothiazide

- **Maxide-25:** 37.5 mg of triamterene and 25 mg of hydrochlorothiazide

- **Moduretic:** 5 mg of amiloride and 50 mg of hydrochlorothiazide

- **Triamterene and Hydrochlorothiazide Capsules and Tablets:** 37.5 mg of triamterene and 25 mg of hydrochlorothiazide

- **Triamterene and Hydrochlorothiazide Tablets:** 75 mg of triamterene and 25 mg of hydrochlorothiazide

- **Triamterene/HCTZ Capsules:** 50 mg of triamterene and 25 mg hydrochlorothiazide

- **Triamterene/HCTZ Capsules and Tablets**: 37.5 mg triamterene and 25 mg hydrochlorothiazide

- **Triamterene/HCTZ Tablets:** 75 mg triamterene and 50 mg hydrochlorothiazide

- **Spironolactone and Hydrochlorothiazide Tablets:** 25 mg spironolactone and 25 mg hydrochlorothiazide

Angiotensin-converting enzyme inhibitors

ACE inhibitors affect the activity of the renin-angiotensin-aldosterone system (see Chapter 4). The body's angiotensin-converting enzyme converts a hormone (angiotensin I) to angiotensin II, which raises blood pressure two ways:

>> It causes direct constriction of arteries.

>> It causes the adrenal gland to release aldosterone, which, in turn, causes salt and water retention.

ACE inhibitors block this enzyme in order to prevent the production of angiotensin II.

In addition to preventing the *increase* in blood pressure, ACE inhibitors also lead to a *decrease* in blood pressure. Angiotensin II breaks down *bradykinen*, a hormone that causes widening of blood vessels. Without angiotensin II, bradykinen levels increase.

TIP

This class of medications has other beneficial side effects, in addition to being a first-line agent for the treatment of high blood pressure. They have heart-protective effects for people diagnosed with heart failure with a decreased ejection fraction. They're also first-line medications for the treatment of kidney disease if there is *proteinuria* (elevated protein in the urine). More than any other drug for high blood pressure, ACE inhibitors slow the progression of these conditions.

Although ACE inhibitors have a number of beneficial effects, their potential side effects include the following:

>> They may lead to elevated potassium levels (especially in patients with heart failure, diabetes, or reduced kidney function) by blocking aldosterone production.

>> They may lead to abnormally low blood pressure if you already have decreased blood volume (for example, after treatment with a diuretic).

>> They may cause a dry cough, which can be very annoying. This can occur at any time while you're taking the medication — even if you've taken the medication for months. If you're on an ACE inhibitor and you develop a dry cough, talk to your doctor.

>> Uncommon side effects include a rash, loss of taste, and reduction of white blood cell count.

WARNING

>> A not-uncommon and serious side effect is *angioneurotic edema*, which causes the throat to swell severely, making it difficult to breathe. Other symptoms of this condition can include lip swelling, tongue swelling, and/or facial swelling, even if you don't have trouble breathing. This is a medical emergency. Call 911.

WARNING

An ACE inhibitor should not be:

>> **Paired with an angiotensin II inhibitor.** This combination can be dangerous because both meds cause increased blood potassium.

>> **Used during pregnancy or in a young woman who plans to become pregnant soon.** ACE inhibitors can adversely affect a growing fetus.

>> **Used during breastfeeding.** They can harm a nursing infant.

Numerous ACE inhibitors are available, and they have some variations in their breakdown. You can recognize them by the *-pril* at the end of their names. Their characteristics are as follows:

>> **Lisinopril (brand names: Prinivil, Zestril):** Lisinopril is probably one of the most commonly prescribed medications for blood pressure in this class. It's very inexpensive and adherence is pretty good because it only needs to be taken once a day. It comes in many strengths: 2.5, 5, 10, 20, 30, and 40 mg. The starting dose is from 2.5 to 40 mg once a day. The kidneys eliminate Lisinopril from the body, so your doctor may decrease your dose if your kidney function is decreased.

Lisinopril also comes with hydrochlorothiazide under the brand name Zestoretic; it contains 10 mg of lisinopril and 12.5 mg of hydrochlorothiazide; 20 mg of lisinopril and 12.5 mg of hydrochlorothiazide; or 20 mg of lisinopril and 25 mg of hydrochlorothiazide. Another medication, with the brand name of Prinzide, contains lisinopril and hydrochlorothiazide in the same proportions.

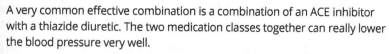

A very common effective combination is a combination of an ACE inhibitor with a thiazide diuretic. The two medication classes together can really lower the blood pressure very well.

>> **Benazepril (brand name: Lotensin):** Benazepril is available as 5-, 10-, 20-, and 40-milligram tablets. It's usually prescribed initially at a dose of 10 mg daily and, if needed, increased to 40 mg once a day or 20 mg twice a day.

Benazepril is also available in combination with hydrochlorothiazide under the brand name Lotensin HCT. The benazepril/ hydrochlorothiazide proportions are: 5 mg/6.25 mg, 10 mg/12.5 mg, 20 mg/12.5 mg, and 20 mg/25 mg.

Benazepril is also packaged as a combination medication with the calcium channel blocker amlodipine under the brand name Lotrel. The amlodipine/ benazepril proportions are 2.5 mg/10 mg, 5 mg/10 mg, and 5 mg/20 mg.

>> **Captopril (brand names: Capoten, Captopril Tablets):** Captopril was the first ACE inhibitor in this class. It comes in 12.5-, 25-, 50-, and 100-milligram strengths and is usually started at 25 mg twice daily; it can be increased up to 150 mg daily divided into two or three doses. Because food decreases the uptake of this drug, it should be taken an hour before meals. Most of the drug is eliminated in the urine, so people with decreased kidney function take less. Captopril seems to cause skin rashes and problems with taste more than the other ACE inhibitors.

Captopril is also sold in a combination with hydrochlorothiazide under the brand name Captopril and Hydrochlorothiazide Tablets. The captopril/hydrochlorothiazide proportions are 25 mg/15 mg, 50 mg/15 mg, 25 mg/25 mg, and 50 mg/25 mg. Some people have trouble with this medication because it's often supposed to be taken two or three times a day.

>> **Enalapril (brand name: Vasotec):** Enalapril comes in 2.5-, 5-, 10-, and 20-milligram tablets. The usual dose is 5 mg once a day increasing to 40 mg once a day or divided into two doses. The kidneys eliminate it, so your doctor will keep you at a lower dose if you have diminished kidney function.

Another medication, with the brand name of Vaseretic, is a combination of enalapril and hydrochlorothiazide. It comes in the following enalapril/hydrochlorothiazide proportions: 5 mg/12.5 mg and 10 mg/25 mg.

Lexxel, another medication, is a combination of enalapril and felodipine (see "Calcium channel blockers," later in this chapter, for more on Lexxel).

>> **Fosinopril (brand name: Monopril):** Fosinopril is available as 10-, 20-, and 40-milligram tablets; it's usually started at 10 mg once a day rising to a maximum of 80 mg a day. If your blood pressure isn't low enough at the end of the single-dose period, you may need to divide the dose so you're taking half the total dosage two times a day. Because fosinopril is broken down in the liver, the usual dose can be given even if you have severe kidney disease.

>> **Moexipril (brand name: Univasc):** Moexipril is available as 7.5- and 15-milligram tablets. The dose usually starts at 7.5 mg once a day at least an hour before a meal. The maximum dose is 30 mg a day, which can be divided into more than one dose. Both liver disease and kidney disease prolong the activity of moexipril, so if you have either of those conditions, your doctor will prescribe a lower amount.

Another medication, with the brand name of Uniretic, is a combination of moexipril and hydrochlorothiazide in the following moexipril/hydro chlorothiazide proportions: 7.5 mg/12 mg and 15 mg/25 mg.

>> **Perindopril (brand name: Aceon):** Perindopril is available in 2-, 4-, and 8-mg tablets. It's usually started at 4 mg and goes up to a maximum of 16 mg once a day. If you have decreased kidney function, your doctor will prescribe a lower dose.

>> **Quinapril (brand name: Accupril):** Quinapril is supplied as 5-, 10-, 20-, and 40-mg tablets. The starting dose is usually 10 mg a day, and the maximum is 80 mg once a day or divided into multiple doses. *Note:* This drug doesn't reach its usual blood levels when taken with a high-fat meal. Because it's eliminated by the kidneys, your doctor will decrease your dose if you have kidney failure.

Another medication, with the brand name Accuretic, is a combination of quinapril and hydrochlorothiazide. The quinapril/ hydrochlorothiazide proportions are 10 mg/12.5 mg, 20 mg/12.5 mg, and 20 mg/25 mg.

» **Ramipril (Altace):** Ramipril is made in 1.25-, 2.5-, 5-, and 10-mg capsules. The dose is usually 2.5 mg to start, and the maximum dose is 20 mg once daily or divided into two doses. Your doctor will decrease your dose if you have kidney disease.

Angiotensin II receptor blockers

Unlike ACE inhibitors (which block the angiotensin-converting enzyme), ARBs don't allow an enzyme to attach to its receptor where the receptor contracts arteries and releases aldosterone. ARBs are necessary because ACE inhibitors aren't effective against other enzymes that make angiotensin II. These receptor blockers, then, can eliminate the activity of angiotensin II more completely. Drugs in this group all end with *–artan.*

Like the ACE inhibitors, ARBs are similar to one another. Advantages of ARBs include the following:

» Like ACE inhibitors, ARBs have a protective effect if you have kidney disease and diabetes and a protective effect if you have heart failure with reduced ejection fraction.

» ARBs can elevate potassium levels, but not to the same degree as ACE inhibitors can.

» ARBs are much less likely to cause a dry cough than ACE inhibitors are.

WARNING

Similar to ACE inhibitors, ARBs shouldn't be prescribed for pregnant or breast-feeding women or women who plan to become pregnant soon.

Some of the medications in this class and their properties are as follows:

» **Candesartan (brand name: Atacand):** Candesartan comes as 4-, 8-, 16-, and 32-mg tablets. The usual starting dose is 16 mg up to a maximum of 32 mg once a day. Your dose won't need to be adjusted if you have mild liver or kidney disease.

Another medication, with the brand name of Atacand-HCT, is a combination of either 16 mg or 32 mg of candesartan and 12.5 mg of hydrochlorothiazide.

» **Eprosartan (brand name: Teveten):** Eprosartan is available as 400- and 600-mg tablets. Starting at 400 mg once daily, the maximum dose is 800 mg once daily. Your dose won't have to be adjusted if you have kidney disease or liver disease.

>> **Irbesartan (brand name: Avapro):** Irbesartan is manufactured as 75-, 150-, and 300-mg tablets. Starting at 150 mg once a day, the dose can go up to 300 mg once a day.

Another medication, with the brand name of Avalide, is a combination of irbesartan and hydrochlorothiazide. The irbesartan/hydrochlorothiazide proportions are 150 mg/12.5 mg or 300 mg/25 mg.

>> **Losartan (brand name: Cozaar):** Losartan was the first member of this class to be approved by the U.S. Food and Drug Administration (FDA). It comes as 25-, 50-, and 100-mg tablets. Treatment usually begins with 50 mg and goes up to 100 mg as a single dose or divided in half and taken twice a day.

TIP

Losartan is a very commonly prescribed blood pressure medication in this class. Not only it is a good blood pressure medication, but it's the only medication in this class that can lower uric acid levels, which makes it very beneficial if you have gout.

Another medication, with the brand name of Hyzaar, is losartan with hydro-chlorothiazide. The losartan/hydrochlorothiazide proportions are 50 mg/12.5 mg, 100 mg/12.5 mg, or 100 mg/25 mg.

>> **Olmesartan (brand name: Benicar):** Olmesartan comes in 5-, 20-, and 40-mg tablets. It's given at a starting dose of 20 mg to a maximum dose of 40 mg once daily.

>> **Telmisartan (brand name: Micardis):** Telmisartan is made in 20-, 40-, and 80-mg tablets. The beginning dose is usually 40 mg once a day up to 80 mg once a day.

Another medication, with the brand name of Micardis HCT, is a combination of telmisartan and hydrochlorothiazide. The telmisartan/hydrochlorothiazide proportions are 40 mg/12.5 mg or 80 mg/25 mg.

>> **Valsartan (Diovan):** Valsartan is produced in 40-, 80-, 160-, and 320-mg capsules. Starting with 80 mg, the dose can go up to 320 mg once a day.

Another medication, Diovan HCT, is valsartan plus hydrochlorothiazide. The valsartan/hydrochlorothiazide proportions are 80 mg/12.5 mg, 160 mg/12.5 mg, 160 mg/25 mg, 320 mg/12.5 mg, and 320 mg/25 mg.

TIP

Health-care providers often think of ACE inhibitors and ARBs interchangeably because they have many of the same properties and same indications. ARBs are a good option if you're unable to tolerate an ACE inhibitor.

Calcium channel blockers

CCBs take advantage of the fact that calcium has to move into the muscle cell in order for a muscle in an artery to contract. These medications block that movement so the muscle can relax. The result is larger arteries and lower blood pressure. So, CCBs act like a vasodilator, but the mechanism is different.

REMEMBER

As arteries widen and peripheral resistance declines, the body responds by increasing the heart rate. Note: This isn't true of all CCBs; some CCBs, particularly verapamil and diltiazem, slow the heart so the heart rate doesn't increase.

TECHNICAL STUFF

Verapamil and diltiazem are CCBs, but they work differently from the medications mentioned next. Although they do have some effect on high blood pressure, they aren't as effective as the medications ending in –*pine*. They're more commonly prescribed by cardiologists to help control a fast heart rate if there is an abnormal heart rhythm present.

Examples of the CCBs commonly prescribed for high blood pressure include the following:

>> **Amlodipine (brand name: Norvasc):** Amlodipine is arguably the most commonly prescribed medication among CCBs for blood pressure control. It also has indications for secondary stroke prevention as well. This medication comes in 2.5-, 5-, and 10-mg tablets. Its initial prescription is usually 5 mg once a day with a maximum of 10 mg once a day. Elderly people usually start at 2.5 mg.

Amlodipine is also sold in combination with benazepril as Lotrel in different strengths. I discuss benazepril in more detail earlier in this chapter.

>> **Felodipine (brand name: Plendil):** Felodipine comes as an extended-release tablet in 2.5-, 5-, and 10-mg strengths. The starting dose is usually 5 mg once a day, and the maximum is 10 mg once a day. It's taken without food or with a light meal and swallowed whole.

Felodipine also comes in combination with enalapril as Lexxel. I discuss enalapril in more detail earlier in this chapter.

>> **Nifedipine (brand names: Adalat Capsules, Procardia Capsules):** Nifedipine is available as 10- or 20-mg capsules. The dose is usually 10 mg three times a day up to 40 mg three times a day. Because of the inconvenience of three daily doses, extended-release formulations (Adalat CC Extended Release Tablets, Procardia XL Extended Release Tablets, and Nifedipine Extended-release Tablets) are available; these come in strengths of 30, 60, and 90 mg.

TIP

Nifedipine is the only CCB that can be used during pregnancy and while breastfeeding.

CCBs have several side effects, but these side effects rarely cause people to stop taking the drug. The main side effects are headache, flushing in the face, dizziness, and swelling of the legs. CCBs may also irritate the stomach and the *esophagus* (the passageway from the mouth to the stomach). Constipation is also common with CCBs as well.

Sustained-release preparations have been developed to try to reduce the side effects, but they may not help with the leg swelling. For some people, the leg swelling is significant enough that the medication needs to be stopped.

Medications that act on the nervous system

The *sympathetic nervous system* (SNS) is the part of the nervous system responsible for increased constriction of the arteries, which raises blood pressure. The SNS uses hormones called *epinephrine* and *norepinephrine* to act as *neurotransmitters* (chemical messengers) along the nerves. Your brain sends out specialized proteins called *neurotransmitters* that transmit a message to that nerve to do something. When the brain wants action, for example, like to cause a blood vessel to narrow, it sends out neurotransmitters that helps to connect the end of one nerve to the beginning of another nerve. Receptors located at the beginning of nerves take up the neurotransmitter so the signal can proceed down the nerve to produce a specific action. It turns out that medications that act on the SNS also can lower blood pressure.

The medications discussed in this section are not first-line agents for high blood pressure, but they have their place in specialized situations.

Methyldopa

Methyldopa (brand names: Aldomet, Methyldopa Tablets) is a medication that acts within the brain to prevent the release of neurotransmitters. It's really only used if other medications don't work or if you're pregnant. Methyldopa is safe during pregnancy, but it isn't the initial choice because of side effects and the fact that it often has to be taken three or four times a day. It can cause anemia, and your doctor will need to monitor your liver function while you're taking it.

The medication can be found in breast milk, but the levels noted are very low. Talk with your doctor if you're breastfeeding.

Methyldopa comes in 125-, 250-, and 500-mg tablets. It usually begins to work in two hours, and its effect lasts about eight hours. Patients usually take a dose of 250 mg three or four times a day; the dosage is raised or lowered every few days until blood pressure control is achieved. The maximum dose is four 500-mg tablets a day. Methyldopa is eliminated from the body through the kidneys for the most part, so if you have reduced kidney function you'll have to take a lower dose.

Clonidine

Clonidine (brand names: Catapres, Clonidine Hydrochloride Tablets, Clonidine HCl Tablets) lowers blood pressure by reducing levels of norepinephrine. This medication is used when other medications don't work, mainly because of its side effects, including the following:

>> **Sleepiness:** Because it can cause sleepiness, you should take it before bed. Dosage increases occur at bedtime.

>> **Dry mouth:** You may find yourself drinking more water to try to counteract this effect.

>> **Depression and disturbing dreams:** The medication may cause depression and vivid dreams or nightmares.

WARNING

Do not stop this medication cold turkey. Stopping this medication, especially if you're taking a higher dose, must be gradual because stopping suddenly may cause withdrawal symptoms, including headaches, shakiness, and a rise in blood pressure *above* the original high level. If you find yourself in a situation where you have to stop taking this medication for any reason (for example, if you must stop taking it before surgery), your doctor will likely substitute another medication well in advance.

Clonidine comes in 0.1-, 0.2-, and 0.3-mg strengths. It's usually prescribed as a starting dose of 0.1 mg two to three times daily and changed on a weekly basis depending on the blood pressure. The maximum dose is usually 0.6 mg, although some doctors use more. It usually begins to act within an hour and lasts for roughly six to eight hours.

Clonidine is also marketed as Catapres-TTS, a patch containing 0.1, 0.2, or 0.3 mg that's applied to the skin. Each patch lasts a week — as long as it doesn't fall off — and it must be replaced at the same time every week.

Beta-adrenergic receptor blockers

Beta-adrenergic receptor blockers, generally known as *beta blockers,* can be used in the treatment of high blood pressure, but they're most commonly used in specialized circumstances:

>> If you've recently had a heart attack

>> If you have heart failure with reduced ejection fraction

Beta blockers can work on two different receptors: beta 1 and beta 2. Beta-1 receptors are found on the heart, and beta-2 receptors are found on the lungs. Some medications in this class block specifically the beta-1 receptor; others also block beta-2 receptors. As the dose of the beta blocker rises, its specificity declines, and the same beta blocker can block both receptors.

Beta blockers are associated with a few side effects, including the following:

>> **Aggravated asthma:** Medications that block beta-2 receptors can aggravate asthma.

>> **Slow heart rate:** Beta blockers can decrease the heart rate.

>> **Fatigue:** Fatigue can be due to the medication's effect on lowering blood pressure or it can be a direct effect of the medication itself.

>> **Increased blood pressure if stopped suddenly:** If you suddenly stop taking a beta blocker, your blood pressure may rebound higher than it was before you started treatment. If you have to stop taking it for any reason, you'll have to do so gradually over a few weeks under the supervision of your doctor.

>> **Lowered blood sugar:** If you have diabetes, beta blockers may blunt the body's response to low blood glucose levels. Very low blood glucose can cause a fast heart rate and tremors to occur that may not show if you're on this medication. If you have diabetes, talk with your doctor before taking a beta blocker.

>> **Slow fetal growth:** You should not take beta blockers during pregnancy because they slow the growth of the fetus.

The following sections review the commonly prescribed beta blockers.

ATENOLOL

Atenolol (brand names: Tenormin, Atenolol Tablets) is available in 25-, 50-, or 100-mg tablets. The starting dose is usually 25 mg once a day up to a maximum of 200 mg once a day.

Atenolol also comes in combination form as Tenoretic 50 (which has 50 mg of atenolol and 25 mg of chlorthalidone) and Tenoretic 100 (which has 100 mg of atenolol and 25 mg of chlorthalidone). Atenolol and Chlorthalidone Tablets are the same two combinations made by another drug company.

Atenolol in any form is eliminated by the kidney. If you have chronic kidney disease, your doctor will need to limit your dose of this medication.

BISOPROLOL

Bisoprolol (brand name: Zebeta) comes in 5- and 10-mg tablets. For high blood pressure, the starting dose is usually 5 mg, but some patients do well with half that dose. The maximum dose is 20 mg once a day. Bisoprolol is eliminated by both the kidneys and the liver, so if you have kidney or liver disease, your doctor will need to lower your medication dosing.

METOPROLOL

Metoprolol (brand names: Lopressor, Metoprolol Tartrate Tablets) comes in 50- and 100-mg strengths. The usual dose is 50 mg twice a day up to a daily maximum dose of 200 mg.

A slow-release form of this drug, Toprol XL, is usually prescribed once a day. It comes in 25-, 50-, 100-, and 200-mg tablets.

Both metoprolol and Toprol XL are eliminated by the liver. If you have liver disease, your doctor will likely need to lower your medication dosing.

NADOLOL

Nadolol (brand names: Corgard, Nadolol Tablets) comes in 20-, 40-, 80-, 120-, and 160-mg tablets. The starting dose is usually 20 mg once a day up to 160 mg once a day.

The kidney is the main site of elimination. If you have kidney disease, your doctor will likely need to lower your medication dosing.

Nadolol also comes in combination with bendroflumethiazide in a medication called Corzide. The nadolol/bendroflumethiazide proportions are 40 mg/5 mg or 80 mg/5 mg.

PROPRANOLOL

Propranolol (brand names: Inderal Tablets, Propranolol Hydrochloride Oral Solution, Propranolol Hydrochloride Tablets) comes in 10-, 20-, 40-, 60-, and 80-mg strengths. The initial prescription is usually 20 mg twice daily up to 160 mg twice daily. This drug was the earliest of the beta blockers, so doctors have the most experience with it.

Propranolol is eliminated by the liver. If you have liver disease, your doctor will likely need to lower your medication dosing.

Propranolol also comes in a long-acting form called Inderal LA (60-, 80-, 120-, or 160-mg strengths) and an extended-release form called InnoPran XL (80- and 120-mg strengths), which allow for once-a-day dosing.

It also comes in combination with hydrochlorothiazide in two different medications: Inderide and Propranolol Hydrochloride. These medications are available in the following propranolol/hydrochlorothiazide proportions: 40 mg/25 mg or 80 mg/25 mg. Finally, a long-acting preparation of Inderide, called Inderide LA, contains 80, 120, or 160 mg of propranolol plus 50 mg of hydrochlorothiazide; it can be taken once a day.

TIP

Propranolol is prescribed as a medication for migraines. If you suffer from migraines, it can kill two birds with one stone by treating your high blood pressure as well preventing migraines.

CARVEDILOL

Carvedilol (brand name: Coreg) comes as 3.125-, 6.25-, 12.5-, and 25-mg tablets. The starting dose is usually 6.25 mg twice daily up to a maximum amount of 25 mg twice daily.

The liver breaks down carvedilol, so if you have liver disease, your doctor will likely need to lower your medication dosing.

REMEMBER

Carvedilol is also used for the treatment of heart failure with reduced ejection fraction. Carvedilol blocks both the alpha and beta receptors and is effective for blood pressure control if first-line agents aren't working.

LABETALOL

Labetalol (brand names: Trandate, Labetalol HCl Tablets) comes as 100-, 200-, and 300-mg tablets. It differs from most of the other beta blockers because of its effect on alpha receptors (see the following section), which then often causes dizziness. The drug has been associated with fever and liver abnormalities. The daily dosage is usually 200 mg divided into two doses up to 1,200 mg divided into two to three doses. The liver is the major organ of elimination.

REMEMBER

Labetalol blocks both the alpha and beta receptors and is effective medications for blood pressure control if first-line agents aren't working.

Alpha-1 adrenergic receptor antagonists

Alpha-1 adrenergic receptor antagonists, known as *alpha blockers,* block another group of sympathetic nerve receptors, some of which are alpha 1 (located in smooth, muscle-like blood vessels) and some of which are alpha 2 (located where nerves connect to each other). Only the alpha-1 blockers are used clinically because they relax muscles in blood vessels to increase the size of the vessel and lower blood pressure. They also lower the bad fats (triglycerides and LDL cholesterol) and raise the good fat (HDL cholesterol).

Alpha blockers are not first-line agents for the treatment of high blood pressure. They're most commonly prescribed for the treatment of high blood pressure and benign prostatic hyperplasia (BPH). A significant side effect of this medication is dizziness on standing. Another effect of this medication is *first-dose phenomenon*, in which the blood pressure drops very low after the first dose or when the drug dose is rapidly increased. This effect is especially common for patients already on a diuretic or a beta blocker. Avoid driving or performing difficult tasks for the first 24 hours after the first dose, which should be taken at bedtime. The effect goes away after the first few doses.

The more commonly prescribed medications in this group include the following:

>> **Doxazosin (brand names: Cardura, Doxazosin):** Doxazosin comes in 1-, 2-, 4-, and 8-mg tablets, with a starting dose of 1 mg at bedtime. The dosage can go up to 16 mg once a day. ***Note:*** Doxazosin is not a good choice during pregnancy. Dizziness and fatigue occur in many people who take it. It's eliminated by the liver. If you have liver disease, your doctor will likely need to lower your medication dosing.

>> **Prazosin (brand names: Minipress, Prazosin HCl Capsules, Prazosin Hydrochloride Capsules, Prazosin HCl Capsules):** Prazosin comes as 1-, 2-, and 5-mg tablets. It's usually taken at a starting dose of 1 mg at bedtime up to 20 mg daily in two or three divided doses. Prazosin isn't recommended for women who are pregnant or breastfeeding.

>> **Terazosin (brand names: Hytrin, Terazosin Capsules, Terazosin Hydrochloride Capsules, Terazosin Tablets):** Terazosin is produced in 1-, 2-, 5-, and 10-mg strengths. The initial daily dose is 1 mg at bedtime increasing to 20 mg divided into two doses if necessary.

Because of their tendency to cause dizziness on standing, these medications are used only when other medications are not effective.

Vasodilators: Medications that open the blood vessels

Vasodilators are drugs that relax the muscles in the arteries, making them larger and reducing blood pressure in the process. When taken alone, these medications can cause an increase in heart rate, depending on the dose. They also can sometimes cause fluid retention and the feeling of a rapid heartbeat. Some vaso-dilators, like nitroglycerin, can cause headaches.

If your doctor needs to prescribe these medications, vasodilators are often taken with diuretics (to help get rid of excess fluid) and beta blockers (to slow the heart). Doctors usually reserve the use of two vasodilators — hydralazine and minoxidil — for the most difficult cases because of their side effects.

Hydralazine

Although hydralazine (brand names: Apresoline, Hydralazine HCl Tablets) was one of the earliest medications prescribed for high blood pressure, it was seldom prescribed because it caused a rapid heart rate and lost its effectiveness after a patient took it for a while (the body compensated for the open blood vessels by increasing the heart rate and retaining water). This medication has only a modest effect on lowering blood pressure, but it is still used for second-line treatment of heart failure for people who are unable to tolerate ACE inhibitors or ARBs. It's also very useful for severe high blood pressure during pregnancy.

WARNING

Hydralazine can also cause a unique drug reaction called lupus-like syndrome after being on the medication for a few months (and more frequently as the dose goes higher). About 50 percent of people break down the drug slowly, and they develop this condition more often than the other 50 percent of people, who break down the drug quickly. The symptoms consist of fever, rash, itching, pain in the joints, and actual swelling, redness, and heat in the joints. After the drug is stopped, the condition usually subsides.

Hydralazine is available in 10-, 25-, 50-, and 100-mg strengths. It's usually taken twice a day and lasts about 12 hours. The maximum dose is 200 mg divided into three to four doses.

Minoxidil

Minoxidil (brand names: Loniten, Minoxidil Tablets) controls the most severe and resistant cases of high blood pressure. Minoxidil relaxes *smooth muscle* (the mus-cle in the walls of arteries) very well and is most useful for severe high blood pres-sure that doesn't respond to other drugs. It's almost always administered with a diuretic and a beta blocker to reverse its undesirable side effects of fluid retention and a fast heart rate.

Minoxidil has been used in children, but it's not recommended for pregnant women or women who are breastfeeding.

Minoxidil increases the workload of the heart. If you have coronary artery disease, your doctor may not prescribe this drug because it increases the workload of the heart. If you have heart failure, your doctor may not prescribe it because this medication tends to cause sodium retention.

Minoxidil can cause increased hair growth on the face, back, arms, and legs after a person is on the drug for several months.

It's available in 2.5- and 10-mg tablets. The starting dose may be as little as 1.25 mg once a day up to a maximum of 40 mg once a day. It begins to work in about 30 minutes.

Choosing the Right Medication

Your doctor will be instrumental in suggesting which medication to use, but your input is important. In this section, I help you go into a conversation with your doctor as a well-informed patient — the kind who can be a partner in your own care.

Reviewing basic principles of medication dosing

When your doctor is prescribing a medication for the treatment of high blood pressure, they'll follow some basic steps:

1. **Ideally, choose a medication that is inexpensive, has minimal side effects, and only needs to be taken once a day.**

   Some doctors prescribe two medications at a smaller dose at the same time if the blood pressure is very elevated at the time of diagnosis (see Chapter 2).

2. **Start with the lowest dose possible.**

   This is especially important for older people because they often take other medications and have other medical conditions, like heart failure, kidney disease, and liver disease.

3. **Increase the dose slowly until the blood pressure goal is achieved.**

4. **If the blood pressure isn't controlled at a reasonable dose, add a second medication that works in a different way.**

5. **If you can't tolerate the initially prescribed medication because of side effects, switch to a medication that works in a different way.**

Arriving at the right medication and the right dosage usually takes some time, so don't be surprised by this process. It's totally normal.

Personalizing the medication choice

Your doctor will consider your other medical conditions when prescribing a medication to lower your blood pressure. Here are some examples:

- >> If you've recently had a heart attack due to coronary artery disease as well as high blood pressure, your doctor will likely suggest a beta blocker and/or an ACE inhibitor.
- >> If you have diabetes with kidney disease along with high blood pressure, your doctor will likely suggest an ACE inhibitor or one of the ARBs.
- >> If you have hand tremors along with high blood pressure, you may respond better to certain beta blockers like propranolol or nadolol.
- >> If you have heart failure, your doctor will probably prescribe an ACE inhibitor and a loop diuretic. Aldosterone antagonists and beta blockers are also prescribed if needed.
- >> If you have heart rhythm abnormalities with high blood pressure, you may do better on beta blockers or CCBs like verapamil or diltiazem (but not CCBs ending in -*pine*).
- >> If you have hyperthyroidism with high blood pressure, you may do best with a beta blocker.
- >> If you have migraine headaches and high blood pressure, you may respond better to certain beta blockers (propranolol or nadolol) or CCBs (verapamil or diltiazem).

Selecting another medication when necessary

If a prescribed medication can't keep your blood pressure consistently under 130/80 mm Hg, your doctor will want to take further action:

- >> If your blood pressure doesn't respond or the side effects are intolerable, they'll prescribe a drug from another medication class. The initial choices are from the first-line agents, including the thiazide diuretics, ACE inhibitors, ARBs, and/or CCBs.

>> If your blood pressure is only partially controlled, a second drug from another medication class can be added. If a thiazide diuretic hasn't been added, it should be added at this point.

>> If your blood pressure still isn't controlled, a third medication can be added.

REMEMBER

Even if you need several medications to bring your blood pressure under control, this doesn't necessarily mean you'll be taking all these drugs the rest of your life. If you're able to incorporate lifestyle changes, you may be able to reduce your medication dosage or even stop some of the medications — with your doctor's blessing, of course.

Adhering to the medication prescription

TIP

What if you have trouble remembering to take your medication every day? Here are some tips to make sure you remember:

>> Pick a time of day when you're always home and take your medication at that time every day.

>> Take your medication at the same time you do another daily task, like brushing your teeth or eating breakfast.

>> If your medication must be taken with food, take it with the same meal every day.

>> Buy a plastic pillbox with a compartment for each day of the week, and fill it at the beginning of every week. That way, you'll be able to see whether you took today's medication.

>> Set an alarm on your phone or use an app (like Medisafe or EveryDose) to remind you to take your pills every day.

WARNING

If you forget to take a dose, don't double the next dose! Just pick up where you left off as though you had taken the medication. If you have any questions regarding a missed dose, don't hesitate to call your doctor.

Recognizing Common Medication Side Effects

Being aware of medication side effects is important. Many blood pressure medications have side effects; some are so severe that people have to stop taking the medication. If you notice an uncomfortable change shortly after you start a new drug for high blood pressure, you may be able to recognize which drug is to blame. But sometimes the side effect doesn't become apparent until months after you start the drug. Other times, the addition of *another* medication (for example, one that's treating another medical condition) may bring out the side effect of the first drug.

Table 13-1 lists common side effects matched with the blood pressure medications that are likely to cause them.

TABLE 13-1

Common Side Effects of Medications

Side Effect	Drug That May Cause It
Anemia	Methyldopa
Breast enlargement	Spironolactone
Confusion	All diuretics
Constipation	CCBs and diuretics
Decreased good cholesterol	Beta blockers
Decreased white blood cells	ACE inhibitors
Depression	Clonidine and CCBs
Diarrhea	Potassium-sparing diuretics and beta blockers
Dizziness	All diuretics, labetalol, and doxazosin
Drowsiness	Alpha blockers and beta blockers
Dry cough	ACE inhibitors
Dry eyes	Clonidine
Dry mouth	All diuretics, methyldopa, and clonidine
Fatigue	Beta blockers and doxazosin
Fever	Methyldopa and labetalol
Fluid in breasts	Methyldopa and spironolactone
Headache	Vasodilators, CCBs, and ACE inhibitors
Heart failure	Alpha-1 adrenergic receptor antagonists and vasodilators
Increased asthma	Beta blockers and diuretics
Increased blood sugar	All diuretics and beta blockers

Side Effect	Drug That May Cause It
Increased cholesterol	Thiazide diuretics
Increased hairiness	Spironolactone and minoxidil
Increased urination	All diuretics and beta blockers
Insomnia and sleep disorders	Beta blockers
Irritation of the esophagus	CCBs
Liver damage	Methyldopa
Loss of hearing	Loop diuretics
Loss of taste	ACE inhibitors
Lupus syndrome	Hydralazine
Menstrual irregularities	Spironolactone
Muscle pains	All diuretics
Nausea and vomiting	All diuretics
Rapid heart rate	Vasodilators
Reduced erections	Thiazide diuretics, spironolactone, and methyldopa
Sensitivity to cold	Alpha blockers and beta blockers
Sensitivity to sunlight	Beta blockers and diuretics
Skin rashes	All diuretics and ACE inhibitors
Sleepiness	Methyldopa and clonidine
Swelling of the abdomen	Potassium-sparing diuretics
Swelling of the legs	Vasodilators and CCBs
Swollen, tender gums	CCBs
Thirst	All diuretics
Upset stomach	Beta blockers, diuretics, and ARBs
Very low blood pressure	ACE inhibitors
Vivid dreams or nightmares	Clonidine and beta blockers
Weakness	All diuretics

If a side effect in this list describes how you're feeling, tell your doctor and ask if you should reduce the dosage or switch to a different class of drugs.

Many other less-common problems are not listed here. If you have an unusual new symptom after starting a drug for high blood pressure, discuss it with your doctor.

In general, medications in the same class have the same side effects. To rid yourself of an annoying side effect, you may have to switch to a new medication class.

Identifying Brand Names

So many medications, so many brand names. How is it possible know what you're taking, much less what it does and what its side effects may be? Doctors often refer to a drug by its brand name because remembering the brand name is easier than remembering the generic name.

In Table 13-2, you can review the brand names of medications in alphabetical order. To find a scientific name, just look up a brand name — its scientific name is in the right-hand column.

Some of these medications are no longer made under their brand name after their patent has run out. If your doctor is still using the brand name, you'll need to know it as well as its generic name.

TABLE 13-2

Brand Names and Their Generic Names

Brand Name	Generic Name
Accupril	Quinapril
Accuretic	Quinapril and hydrochlorothiazide
Aceon	Perindopril
Adalat	Nifedipine
Aldactone	Spironolactone
Aldomet	Methyldopa
Altace	Ramipril
Apresoline	Hydralazine

Brand Name	Generic Name
Atacand	Candesartan
Avalide	Irbesartan and hydrochlorothiazide
Avapro	Irbesartan
Benicar	Olmesartan
Bumex	Bumetanide
Capoten	Captopril
Cardura	Doxazosin
Catapres	Clonidine
Corgard	Nadolol
Coreg	Carvedilol
Corzide	Nadolol and bendroflumethiazide
Cozaar	Losartan
Demadex	Torsemide
Diovan	Valsartan
Diovan HCT	Valsartan and hydrochlorothiazide
Dyazide	Triamterene and hydrochlorothiazide
Dyrenium	Triamterene
Edecrin	Ethacrynic acid
HydroDIURIL	Hydrochlorothiazide
Hytrin	Terazosin
Hyzaar	Losartan and hydrochlorothiazide
Inderal	Propranolol
Inderide	Propranolol and hydrochlorothiazide
InnoPran XL	Propranolol
Lasix	Furosemide
Lexxel	Felodipine and enalapril
Loniten	Minoxidil
Lopressor	Metoprolol

(continued)

TABLE 13-2 *(continued)*

Brand Name	Generic Name
Lotensin	Benazepril
Lotrel	Amlodipine and benazepril
Maxide	Triamterene and hydrochlorothiazide
Midamor	Amiloride
Minipress	Prazosin
Micardis	Telmisartan
Micardis HCT	Telmisartan and hydrochlorothiazide
Moduretic	Amiloride and hydrochlorothiazide
Monopril	Fosinopril
Mykrox	Metolazone
Norvasc	Amlodipine
Prinzide	Lisinopril and hydrochlorothiazide
Procardia	Nifedipine
Teveten	Eprosartan
Thalitone	Chlorthalidone
Toprol XL	Metoprolol
Trandate	Labetalol
Uniretic	Moexipril and hydrochlorothiazide
Univasc	Moexipril
Vasotec	Enalapril
Zaroxolyn	Metolazone
Zebeta	Bisoprolol
Zestril	Lisinopril
Zestoretic	Lisinopril and hydrochlorothiazide

Chapter **14**

Considering Important Clinical Studies of High Blood Pressure

Since the last version of this book, some landmark clinical studies have changed how doctors treat high blood pressure. Today, doctors recognize that the lower the blood pressure, even in older people, the lower the risk of heart attack and stroke. The ultimate goal is to reduce the end organ effects of high blood pressure (discussed in Part 2 of this book).

REMEMBER

Two of the major aspects that have changed regarding the approach and treatment of high blood pressure have been a recognition of the genetic component of high blood pressure (see Chapter 3) and lowering the blood pressure goals.

Doctors know the many dangers of uncontrolled high blood pressure. Their goal is to use the best clinical evidence available to talk with you about treatment options. Recently, newer blood pressure guidelines have come out, with new classifications of blood pressure, new guidelines about medications for high blood pressure, and new goals for what blood pressure should be (see Chapter 2).

TIP

When doctors review clinical research studies, we pay attention to the following when interpreting the results:

>> Who was enrolled in the study? What is their age and gender? What other medical conditions do they have?

>> Did the study have enough people enrolled so that the results of the study can be applied to the population as a whole?

>> Were there any important exclusion criteria for the individuals in the study? For example, in the SPRINT trial (covered in the next section), people with diabetes were not included in the study, but many people with diabetes also have high blood pressure.

This chapter provides a brief overview of several major clinical studies that your doctor will be aware of when treating your high blood pressure.

SPRINT: Systolic Blood Pressure Intervention Trial

One of the ways scientists show how cool they are is by naming their trials with awesome acronyms. The Systolic Blood Pressure Intervention Trial (known as SPRINT) was a clinical research study that evaluated more than 9,000 people (that's a lot!) aged 50 years or older with systolic blood pressure readings between 130 mm Hg and 180 mm Hg (systolic is the top number). The goal was to evaluate the effects of lowering the systolic blood pressure to less than 120 mmHg in one group compared to lowering the blood pressure to less than 140 mmHg in the other group.

When I say "effects," what am I referring to? The study looked at the end organ effects of high blood pressure, including heart attack, heart failure, stroke, and death to due heart disease. The results of the SPRINT study were striking: Risk of heart attack, stroke, heart failure, and death due to heart disease decreased by 25 percent in the group in which the systolic blood pressure was lowered to less than 120 mm Hg. Death from *any cause* was also decreased in this group.

People in this group also seemed to be able to tolerate the lowered blood pressure. One significant aspect of the study was that there was no significant difference in *orthostatic blood pressures* (lowered blood pressure with going from a sitting to standing position) in different positions between the two different groups. There was a slight increase in the risk of acute kidney injury in the lower treatment group, but it wasn't as significant as doctors would expect.

So, what is the effect of this study in terms of how doctors approach blood pressure in middle-aged adults and older adults? Doctors are now trying to get systolic blood pressure down to at least 130/80 mm Hg in their older patients, or 120/80 mm Hg if they're able to tolerate that.

TECHNICAL STUFF

People with diabetes and stroke were excluded from this study. This is important because diabetes is a very common condition affecting millions and it increases stroke risk and is commonly seen with high blood pressure. Stroke is a known complication of high blood pressure. Excluding people with these medical conditions means that the results of this study can't just be recognized as recommendations for everyone with high blood pressure.

STEP: Strategy of Blood Pressure Intervention in the Elderly Hypertensive Patients

Although the SPRINT trial (covered in the preceding section) noted that a systolic blood pressure goal of less than 120 mm Hg systolic reduced the risk of heart attack, stroke, heart failure, and death due to heart disease, there remained a concern as to how well older patients would tolerate a lowering of blood pressure. Older people in general have a greater risk of falling and dizziness, and the concern was that lower blood pressure might increase this risk. In addition, as noted in Chapter 2, blood pressure measurements may vary from an office blood pressure reading to one taken at home. Measuring blood pressure at home is very important for getting a better sense of someone's true blood pressure. Thus, the STEP trial.

STEP stands for Strategy of Blood Pressure Intervention in the Elderly Hypertensive Patients. In this study, 8,000 participants were divided into two groups; one group of patients had a systolic blood pressure goal of 110 mm Hg to 129 mm Hg, and the other group of patients had a systolic blood pressure goal of 130 mm Hg to 149 mm Hg. The participants were all Chinese people ages 60 to 80 with a history of high blood pressure. To be able to be included in the study, they had have a systolic blood pressure between 140 m Hg and 190 mm Hg. People with a history of a stroke could not participate in the study, but people with diabetes were included. The individuals in the study underwent regular follow-up for a period of four years. Their blood pressure was measured with a validated (see Chapter 2) automated blood pressure monitor. Blood pressures were also measured in the office using an automated blood pressure cuff using a specific protocol in which the patients had to sit for several minutes (see Chapter 2).

The results of the trial demonstrated that people in the treatment group with a lower blood pressure goal of 110 mm Hg to 129 mm Hg had a significant reduction in cardiac events and stroke compared to those whose blood pressure goal was 130 mm Hg to 149 mm Hg.

What does this study mean when it comes to how your doctor will treat you? STEP recognizes the importance of home blood pressure monitoring to really get a sense of how someone's blood pressure is doing, so your doctor will likely encourage you to monitor your blood pressure at home. STEP also emphasizes the importance of trying for a lower blood pressure goal (if you haven't had a stroke), so assuming you haven't had a stroke, your doctor may work with you to get your systolic blood pressure below 130 mm Hg.

ACCORD: Action to Control Cardiovascular Risk in Diabetes

The Action to Control Cardiovascular Risk in Diabetes (ACCORD) trial involved more than 10,000 participants all of whom had type 2 diabetes. Everyone in the study received either strict glucose control or standard glucose control. Approximately half of the individuals in this study also received treatment for hyperlipidemia (high cholesterol and/or triglycerides) and approximately a little less than 5,000 of the participants received either strict blood pressure control or less-strict blood pressure control.

To qualify for the study, people had to be 40 years of age or older, have a hemoglobin A1C of 7.5 and have risk factors for heart disease. The strict blood pressure treatment group had a systolic blood pressure goal of less than 120 mm Hg, and the other group's goal was less than 140 mm Hg. Blood pressure follow-up was every month for the first four months with office blood pressure measurements, and then every two months thereafter. In the standard treatment group, the follow-up was less frequent.

The ACCORD study showed that there was no benefit in the intensive treatment group in reducing cardiovascular outcome or mortality rate from any cause. Those in the intensive treatment group had increased risk of adverse events including low potassium levels and risk of worsening kidney function compared to the standard treatment group. People in the more intensely treated group had fewer strokes and cardiac events than those in the other treatment group.

What does this study mean for you? If you have diabetes, controlling your blood pressure is very important. Further studies are ongoing regarding to what the optimal blood pressure is for people with diabetes; the goal should be 130/80 mm Hg or lower, and your doctor should closely monitor your blood pressure.

ADVANCE: Action in Diabetes and Vascular Disease

The Action in Diabetes and Vascular Disease (ADVANCE) trial studied approximately 11,000 people with diabetes and heart disease or a risk factor for heart disease. There were two treatment groups in this study:

>> One group had intense blood glucose control.

>> The other group has less intense blood glucose control.

In addition, one group was treated for blood pressure with perindopril (an ACE inhibitor) plus indapamide (a diuretic) and the other group received a placebo. The people in this study were followed for four and a half years. There were fewer deaths and cardiac events among those in the more intense blood pressure treatment group compared to the placebo group. Controlled blood pressure was defined as a systolic blood pressure of less than 140 mm Hg.

What does this study mean for you? As noted in the preceding section, if you have diabetes, controlling your blood pressure is very important. Your blood pressure goal should be 130/80 mm Hg or lower, and your doctor should close monitor your blood pressure.

4

Taking Care of Special Populations

Chapter **15**

Handling High Blood Pressure in Older Adults

Who are older people? It's a moving definition because people are living longer and longer, but for the purposes of this chapter, older people are 65 or older. When you're older, managing blood pressure is very complex for several reasons:

» You may have more than one medical condition.

» You may take multiple medications, which increases your risk of interactions among the medications.

» You may not be getting proper nutrition.

» Your kidneys may not be functioning well.

» You're at increased risk of stroke and heart attack.

TIP

If you can get your blood pressure to less than 120/80 mm Hg, you'll have a significant reduction in your risk of heart attack and stroke (and dying in general). At the end of the day, however, your blood pressure goal needs to be personalized and tailored to *you*, based on your age, your other medical conditions, and your own wishes regarding your care. This is called *shared decision making*, and it's about you and your health-care provider working together as a team to achieve the best blood pressure possible. Many health-care providers want their older patients to have for a blood pressure of less than 130/80 to reduce the risk of heart attack and stroke.

In this chapter, I fill you in on factors that are important in deciding what your blood pressure goal should be, as well as the intensity of treatment that's right for you.

WARNING

Older people can be very susceptible to lower blood pressures when standing up. This condition is called *orthostatic hypotension* (see Chapter 2), and it can manifest as dizziness, lightheadedness, a fall, worsening tiredness, and/or confusion (an altered mental status due to lowered blood pressure — the brain is not getting the blood pressure it needs). This is an important aspect that would affect the person's blood pressure goal — it may need to be on the higher side to prevent worsening blood pressure and increased symptoms when standing up.

Evaluating Cognitive Ability

An important aspect of consideration is evaluation an individual's cognitive function. Not every older person experiences cognitive decline, but if a question exists about a person's ability to take medications in a timely manner, as well as safely perform the activities of daily living, then evaluating their cognitive ability is important. This step can be a brief mental-status examination by a health-care provider to evaluate the following abilities:

>> Orientation in time (day and year) and space (city and state)

>> Ability to repeat items, read, write, draw, calculate, name items, and remember items previously named

>> Comprehension

Standard versions of this test give an individual score; a perfect score is 30. One version is the Mini Mental State Examination (MMSE), which takes only ten minutes. A person who scores less than 26 probably has some cognitive impairment that can be further tested. This is a good baseline test for any older person, not just for people with high blood pressure, and it can be repeated at intervals to observe a decrease in their mental acuity from baseline. The test can also help determine whether a loss of mental acuity is due to medication, especially if it's performed after a new medication has been introduced and there is a decrease in the score when compared to prior testing.

TIP

Another very commonly used test is the Montreal Cognitive Assessment (MoCA), which assesses for cognitive impairment. Health-care professionals need to undergo training on this assessment before performing it.

Assessing Blood Pressure in an Older Person

In the highly industrialized countries of the world, the populations' systolic blood pressure rises throughout their lives. In contrast, the diastolic blood pressure begins to level off from age 50 to 60, and it often decreases after that. This decrease in the diastolic blood pressure (the bottom number) is due to the result of increasing stiffness of arteries with aging. (See Chapter 2 for a review of systolic and diastolic blood pressure.)

This section covers factors to consider regarding the blood pressure itself in an older person.

Recognizing baseline high blood pressure

Just about all high blood pressure in older people is *essential* — high blood pressure for which the cause is undetermined. (There is nothing essential about high blood pressure, except the terminology!)

Most of the high blood pressure in older people is also *isolated systolic high blood pressure* (where the systolic blood pressure is over 140 mm Hg, but the diastolic blood pressure is less than 90 mm Hg). In older people, increased systolic blood pressure can increase the risk of a stroke or heart attack. In contrast, their diastolic blood pressure elevation doesn't have the same risks as it does in a younger person.

Most often, *isolated diastolic high blood pressure* (where the systolic blood pressure is less than 140 mm Hg, but the diastolic blood pressure is greater than 90 mm Hg) poses no risk among older people. *Note:* A person with isolated diastolic high blood pressure will likely require some treatment, especially when complications of high blood pressure are present.

TIP

If you or a loved one or family member is over 65 years with a systolic blood pressure reading that's greater than 130 on several occasions, talk to your health-care provider for further evaluation and discussion.

DETECTING PSEUDO HIGH BLOOD PRESSURE

Pseudo high blood pressure is a condition resulting from the calcification of the arteries. Due to aging, calcium begins to deposit along the artery and can lead to an inaccurate blood pressure reading (the artery doesn't compress when the cuff around the arm is inflated). Even though the blood pressure inside the artery is normal, the blood pressure meter registers high (as much as 20 to 30 mm Hg higher than its true value). A few clues can indicate this condition:

- No other signs of a high blood pressure complication
- Little change in blood pressure despite adequate treatment
- Low blood pressure symptoms despite normal or even high measured blood pressure

A health-care provider can use other techniques to get a direct measurement of blood pressure to evaluate the possibility of pseudo high blood pressure.

Considering resistant high blood pressure

Resistant high blood pressure means the high blood pressure is a direct result of another condition that is raising the blood pressure. If that other condition causing the elevation in blood pressure goes away or is treated, then the blood pressure usually lowers. (Chapter 4 covers the various causes of resistant high blood pressure.)

An older person's high blood pressure is rarely due to another acute medical condition, but you should consider the possibility of it under the following circumstances:

- ❱❱ The person has newly developed high blood pressure after 60 years of age.
- ❱❱ Three or more blood pressure medications have failed to control the blood pressure.
- ❱❱ Symptoms or lab findings suggest resistant high blood pressure (see Chapter 4 for more on this subject).
- ❱❱ The person has a low potassium level before taking medications or when they take a small dose of a *thiazide diuretic* (see Chapter 13 for more on this type of drug).
- ❱❱ There is continuing evidence of worsening kidney function despite adequate blood pressure control.

The steps to evaluate and treat someone for resistant high blood pressure are discussed in detail in Chapter 4. Resistant high blood pressure in older people may not decrease even when the underlying cause is treated because

>> The high blood pressure may have been present for a long time.

>> Older people also tend to have underlying essential high blood pressure.

Examining the medications that raise blood pressure

Many older people deal with chronic, sometimes debilitating arthritis on a daily basis, the most common cause being "wear and tear" on the joints over the years due to osteoarthritis. The most commonly prescribed treatment for this pain is *nonsteroidal anti-inflammatory drugs* (NSAIDs). Over-the-counter NSAIDs include ibuprofen (with the brand names Advil and Motrin), naproxen (with the brand name Aleve), and aspirin. A variety of NSAIDs are taken by prescription, too.

REMEMBER

The problem is, NSAIDs can raise blood pressure because they cause sodium and water retention. They also can reduce the blood-pressure-lowering effects of any blood pressure medications you may be taking, including thiazide or thiazide-like diuretics (see Chapter 13).

WARNING

If you're taking a low-dose aspirin and you're also taking another NSAID for osteoarthritis, it may increase your bleeding risk, especially from the gastrointestinal tract.

TIP

Arthritis-related pain can be debilitating and affect your quality of life, so if you're dealing with high blood pressure, an option to discuss with your health-care provider is the use of topical Voltaren. You can get it by prescription or over the counter. It is applied four times a day and provides pain relief. It will be absorbed into the bloodstream a bit, but a lot less than if you take the oral form of the medication.

Improving Nutrition to Lower Blood Pressure

When you're older, the goal of nutrition is to provide the right amount of calories with enough nutrients, vitamins, and minerals from the appropriate energy sources. In Chapter 15, I explain the importance of nutrition in the treatment and prevention of high blood pressure. This doesn't change as you get older — in fact, your doctor will probably pay even more attention to your nutritional status to make sure you're getting the nutrition you need.

REMEMBER

Read food labels, especially sodium content, when shopping. Many canned soups, for example, though economical, have a very high sodium content.

Assessing your nutritional status

A nutritional assessment helps to determine if an older person is getting enough of the right foods. One way to assess your nutritional status from a food perspective is to keep a food diary of what you've eaten over a three- to five-day period. Your health-care provider may also order lab tests to help get a better sense of your nutritional status.

TIP

In anyone, but especially an older person, an objective way to follow a person's nutritional status is to track their weight. If you can stand on a scale, weigh yourself the same time every day, or at least a couple times a week, and record your weight. Unintentional weight loss can be a sign of poor nutritional status.

If you're losing weight unintentionally, the weight loss can affect a lot of things. You may be more prone to side effects from medications, including dizziness and lightheadedness from blood-pressure-lowering medications. Unintentional weight loss should be taken seriously and your health-care provider should evaluate you if this is happening.

REMEMBER

A significant factor that also needs to be considered in the assessment of nutritional status are social determinants of health (see Chapter 3). The following factors are very important to consider, especially in older people:

>> Do you drive or have access to reliable transportation to get to your medical appointments and/or to the pharmacy to pick up your medications? Can you afford your medications?

>> What is your baseline functional status? Can you walk without assistance? Are you able to participate in some exercise at home?

>> Do you have access to healthy food? Can you afford healthy food?

>> Do you live alone? Do you have a support system?

Your doctor may ask you the following when assessing your nutritional status:

>> What vitamins and/or other over-the-counter supplements are you currently taking?

>> How many fresh vegetables and fresh fruits do you eat every day?

>> Do you eat a variety of different foods?

>> How much salt are you eating every day?

>> How many calories are you eating every day?

>> Are you able to walk by yourself or do you need a cane or walker to help you?

>> Have you had any recent falls? If you have fallen, were you able to get up by yourself or did you need help?

Following the DASH nutrition plan

Older people who follow the DASH nutrition plan (see Chapter 9) may find that their blood pressure comes down. They may be able to reduce the dosage of their current blood pressure medication or even discontinue a medication. (Don't stop taking your blood pressure medication without talking to your doctor.) The DASH nutrition plan also decreases the risk of heart attack and stroke.

Reducing salt intake

If you're older, minimizing your salt intake is key, because older people tend to be more sensitive to the blood-pressure-raising effects of salt. When you follow the DASH diet *and* you reduce your salt intake, the result is even greater.

WARNING

Reducing salt intake can be especially difficult for older people for a few reasons:

>> Taste sensation can decrease as we get older, so older people may compensate by adding more salt to food. One way to get around this is to use more herbs and spices in place of salt.

>> Older people may live alone and not be able to eat fresh food before it spoils. As a result, they may rely on prepared foods that contain salt. If this sounds familiar, pay closer attention to food labels and look for prepared foods that are low in sodium.

>> Older people may lack the energy or ability to put together a healthy meal. If this is the case for you, invite family and friends over for a meal and have everyone bring a healthy dish to eat.

Modifying Your Lifestyle to Lower Blood Pressure

Lifestyle modifications can really help lower blood pressure in older people. Important lifestyle changes include the following:

>> Reducing or even eliminating your consumption of alcohol (see Chapter 11)

>> Quitting tobacco (see Chapter 11)

>> Reducing excessive caffeine intake (more than two cups of regular coffee per day; see Chapter 11)

>> Increasing daily exercise (see Chapter 12)

>> Adding yoga, meditation, or biofeedback (see Chapter 12)

Lifestyle changes can reduce or even eliminate the need for medications. Don't underestimate the importance of these interventions.

Taking Prescription Medications to Lower Blood Pressure

Chapter 13 does a deep dive into the various classes of medications to lower blood pressure, but there are specific considerations for older people:

>> Thiazide diuretics are commonly prescribed for high blood pressure, but older people, especially older women, are at a higher risk of developing *hyponatremia* (low sodium level). Your doctor can measure your sodium level with a routine blood test. When a person's sodium level is too low, it can cause weakness and an altered mental status. Not eating enough and low body mass index (BMI) are risk factors for the development of hyponatremia.

>> If you have chronic kidney disease and you have to take a loop diuretic (see Chapter 13) such as furosemide to help with fluid management to avoid swelling, your doctor will need to adjust the dose of the diuretic to minimize the risk that you'll have to get up several times at night to use the bathroom. When you're older, if you have to walk to the bathroom at night when it's dark, you're more likely to trip and fall.

>> Your doctor may want to keep you on a once-daily medication instead of a medication you have to take multiple times a day. That way, you're more likely to stick to the routine.

>> When you first start taking a blood pressure medication, your doctor will likely have you start with half the usual beginning dose and then make changes slowly as you get used to the medication.

>> Make sure you can open the medication bottle and you know how to take the medication. Some safety bottles are impossible to open if you have arthritis or vision problems — work with your doctor and/or pharmacist to get that sorted so you don't risk taking the wrong medication at the wrong time.

>> If you can stand and walk, orthostatic blood pressure measurements (see Chapter 2) should be obtained whenever you go for a medical office visit and/ or at home if possible. These should also be done if there is an increase in the dose of an existing medication or if a new medication is being prescribed. If your blood pressure decreases as you stand up, you're at increased risk of falling.

>> Medication interactions are a major potential problem because older people may be taking a number of prescription drugs. Talk with your doctor to try to reduce the number of medications you take.

TIP

When an older person has chest pain due to heart disease, recent heart attack, or heart failure, a beta blocker is a great choice for treating high blood pressure (see Chapter 5). ACE inhibitors have been shown to prolong the lives of people with congestive heart failure — they're the drugs of choice when heart failure accompanies high blood pressure. ACE inhibitors and angiotensin II receptor blockers are especially good for older people with high blood pressure and kidney disease (often associated with diabetes).

Avoiding Dangerous Falls in Blood Pressure

Older people have significant risk of a sudden, dramatic fall in blood pressure when they stand up. When the elderly have systolic high blood pressure, diabetes, or adrenal gland failure, the frequency of these large falls in blood pressure upon standing is even greater. When changing positions (usually from sitting to standing), they can develop symptoms including blurred vision, lightheadedness, dizziness, and even a loss of consciousness.

Two tendencies account for this issue in older people:

>> Blood tends to remain in the lower part of the body because of a loss of muscle tone and a loss of valves in blood vessels that ordinarily prevent blood backflow.

>> Older people sometimes lose the normal response of certain pressure sensors in the neck that detect falling blood pressure. When these sensors are functioning properly, they signal the heart to pump more blood into the brain. The heart pumps harder, and other blood vessels constrict to push blood back to the heart. But when the sensors aren't functioning, the decreased blood in the brain may lead to a fainting spell or dizziness.

TIP

There are a number of approaches for treating falls in blood pressure upon standing, including the following:

>> **Tilt your bed to elevate your head.** If you have diabetes, you may have *autonomic neuropathy,* in which, when you lie down flat, your blood pressure can elevate. Raising the head of the bed can reduce your blood pressure when lying down and minimize the difference in blood pressure when you sit up and/or stand up.

>> **Wear compression socks.** They reduce the pooling of blood in the legs and help to improve the blood flow back to the heart.

>> **Perform leg exercises to push blood back to the heart.** For example, something as simple as walking not only improve the muscle tone in your legs but also helps to improve the efficiency of the blood flowing back to the heart. Other examples of exercises include bicycling and strength training. For an example of exercises that can improve your muscle strength, endurance, and heart health check out https://tools.silversneakers.com.

>> **Ask your doctor if you could be dehydrated.** If so, talk to your doctor about avoiding thiazide diuretics unless absolutely necessary.

>> **Ask your doctor if they can reduce the dose of your blood pressure medication, particularly beta blockers and alpha blockers.**

Chapter **16**

Handling High Blood Pressure in Children

High blood pressure is not just a problem in adults; it's also a problem in kids. According to the Centers for Disease Control and Prevention (CDC), approximately 1 in 25 children ages 12 to 19 have high blood pressure, and this number is only increasing. A significant aspect contributing to the increasing rate of high blood pressure in kids is the increase in childhood obesity. The number of kids with obesity is increasing; according to the CDC, approximately 20 percent of kids ages 2 to 19 are obese.

TIP

A child is considered *overweight* if they're heavier than 85 percent of the children of the same age and height. The child is *obese* if they're heavier than 95 percent of kids of the same age and height. Your child's doctor can talk to you about their weight.

This chapter reviews information you need to help prevent high blood pressure in your child or treat it if your child already has it. (For the purposes of this chapter, children range in age from newborn to age 18.)

TIP

When dealing with high blood pressure or other medical conditions in children, the effects of positive reinforcement on your child can be significant in helping them adhere to their treatment regimen. Rewarding, praising, and encouraging your child's positive efforts are really important!

Measuring Blood Pressure and Interpreting the Results

Just as in adults, proper measurement of a child's blood pressure is essential to make a correct diagnosis. It's generally recommended that kids first have their blood pressure checked at the age of 3. If your child has other medical conditions (for example, any evidence of kidney disease or a significant family history of high blood pressure or heart conditions at a very young age), their blood pressure may have to be measured earlier than this.

Measuring a blood pressure in a child can be especially challenging when they don't really want to have their arm wrapped in a cuff and squeezed. The following sections show you how to get a proper blood pressure reading in any child. Turn to Chapter 2 for the basics of measuring blood pressure.

Taking a blood pressure reading on tiny arms

There are many similarities between measuring blood pressure in children and adults. Just as there are automated blood pressure devices for adults (see Chapter 2) to take their blood pressure at home, there are automated blood pressure machines to measure a child's blood pressure at home.

REMEMBER

Don't rely on the blood pressure measurements taken once a year in the doctor's office, especially if your child has high blood pressure or is at risk of developing high blood pressure. Take measurements at home regularly — at least once a week.

The width of the blood pressure cuff must be appropriate for the size of the child's arm. If the cuff is too small, the reading will be too high; if the cuff is too large, the reading will be too low. The cuff has to completely surround the upper arm, but the length of the *bladder* (the part of the cuff that inflates with air) must also cover at least 80 percent of the circumference of the upper arm. Its width should also be 40 percent of the distance from the elbow to the shoulder.

TIP

If your child is between cuff sizes, use the larger cuff. A small cuff often produces a falsely elevated reading, but a larger cuff usually doesn't change the reading enough to miss a high blood pressure reading.

TIP

To take your child's blood pressure, have them child sit in a chair, with both feet on the floor and their legs uncrossed. Have them place their arm level with their heart. If your child is tall enough, you may be able to do this sitting at the kitchen table. If their feet don't reach the ground sitting at the kitchen table, try having them sit at a child's desk or play table instead — you may have to get a little creative to find the right setup. Try putting a box or crate under their feet if their feet don't touch the ground.

Interpreting the results of the measurement

Children begin their lives with much lower blood pressure than they have later on. The blood pressure range of a newborn can be anywhere from 55/30 mm Hg to 70/45 mm Hg. Within a month, the blood pressure increases to a range of 70/40 mm Hg to 95/60 mm Hg, and the blood pressure continues to rise throughout childhood.

The definition of high blood pressure is different for children under the age of 13 is different than it is for kids 13 and older (and adults). The blood pressure value that defines high blood pressure for kids under 13 is based on *percentiles. High* blood pressure is at or above the 95th percentile; *elevated blood pressure* is from the 90th to 94 percentile. Table 16-1 shows the 95th percentile blood pressure — that is, the maximum normal blood pressures for different ages (under the age of 13).

TABLE 16-1

Maximum Normal Blood Pressure at Different Ages

Age	Blood Pressure
Newborn	70/45 mm Hg
1–5 years	110/75 mm Hg
6–12 years	120/75 mm Hg

TIP

The National Heart, Lung, and Blood Institute has guidelines for the 90th and 95th percentile blood pressure levels for boys and girls ages 1 through 17 at various heights. You can find these guidelines at www.nhlbi.nih.gov/files/docs/guidelines/child_tbl.pdf. If your child has a blood pressure between the 90th percentile and 94th percentile, their blood pressure should be rechecked and you should talk with their doctor about home blood pressure monitoring.

For kids 13 years or older, Table 16-2 outlines how high blood pressure is defined. Systolic blood pressure is the upper number, and diastolic blood pressure is the lower number. For example, in the blood pressure measurement of 120/80, the systolic number if 120 and the diastolic number is 80.

TABLE 16-2	Blood Pressure in Kids 13 and Older		
Category	Systolic Blood Pressure (in mm Hg)		Diastolic Blood Pressure (in mm Hg)
Normal	Less than 120	and	Less than 80
Elevated blood pressure	120–129	and	Less than 80
High blood pressure, stage 1	130–139	and	80–89
High blood pressure, stage 2	140 or greater	and	90 or greater

REMEMBER

Can children have white-coat high blood pressure? Absolutely. A January 2019 article from the journal *Hypertension* suggests that as many as half of all kids may have elevated blood pressure due to the white-coat effect. This is another reason to talk with your child's doctor about home blood pressure monitoring.

Considering the Causes of Elevated Blood Pressure

The causes of high blood pressure in kids can vary, but health conditions that run in families play a significant role. Some factors such as a family history of high blood pressure can help identify kids who are at high risk for developing high blood pressure as adults. The earlier you can take preventive measures, the more likely your child will *not* develop high blood pressure, regardless of the cause. The future of quality high blood pressure care lies in prevention.

Surveying hereditary influences

Genetics undoubtedly influences the development of high blood pressure. If a parent has high blood pressure, their children are more likely to develop high blood pressure. If both parents have high blood pressure, the chances of the children developing high blood pressure increase even more.

Kids who are likely to have high blood pressure as adults because their parents have high blood pressure may react differently to many challenges than kids whose parents *don't* have high blood pressure. For example, kids born to parents with high blood pressure may

>> Have a greater rise in pulse rate than usual during exercise

>> Experience an excessive rise in blood pressure after exercise

>> Respond to emotional stress with a much greater rise in blood pressure

>> Respond to a mental challenge like a school test with a rise in blood pressure

>> Often have increased *plasma renin activity* (increased presence of a chemical that tends to increase blood pressure)

Factoring in weight

A strong relationship between weight and blood pressure exists at any age, but being overweight or obese during childhood is a significant risk factor for high blood pressure early in life and in the child's future. Consider these additional facts:

>> Newborns who have a low birth weight tend to have higher blood pressures by the time they're adolescents than those who have normal weight at birth.

>> If an overweight child loses weight, they often reverse their high blood pressure.

>> Even when the overweight condition doesn't continue into adulthood, an adult who was overweight as a child is at increased risk of developing heart disease as an adult.

Evaluating other possible causes

When a newborn or a child up through 6 years of age has high blood pressure, it's usually *secondary* high blood pressure (the result of another disease). The most common causes in this age group are kidney disease, blockage of one or both arteries to the kidney, or narrowing of the aorta. If your child's blood pressure is elevated — especially if your child is really young — their doctor will look for potential causes like these.

An important clue to the cause of high blood pressure in older kids is the abuse of drugs like amphetamines and cocaine. Vaping may also be associated with an increased risk of developing of high blood pressure.

Initiating Treatment with Lifestyle Changes

Lifestyle changes can control high blood pressure in kids — and these changes may be all that's necessary to reverse the condition, especially in older children. Here are some lifestyle changes you'll want to work on with your child:

>> **Managing stress:** If stress is playing a role in your child's high blood pressure, you'll need to help them manage their stress. You may need to send them for therapy or counseling to help them find tools and techniques for stress management. Or you may be able to help your child yourself by establishing a daily meditation routine with an app like Headspace (www.headspace.com), which has kid-specific meditations.

>> **Choosing healthy foods:** If your child is younger, you're likely in full control of their diet. The older your kid gets, the less control you'll have over what they eat. No matter how old your child is, you can encourage them to follow a diet that is low in fats and has more servings of fruits, vegetables, and grains by eating that way yourself. The DASH diet (see Chapter 9) lowers blood pressure in kids as well as adults.

>> **Controlling diabetes:** If your child has diabetes, controlling their blood glucose can help control their blood pressure.

>> **Exercising:** Exercise (see Chapter 12) is another key to dealing with high blood pressure. Kids need to understand that moving their bodies is just as important to their health as eating properly. Try to help your kid find an exercise that they enjoy — this will increase the likelihood that they'll stick with the exercise regimen. Plus, if they can do the exercise or activity with friends, they're more likely to continue it. Sticking your kid on a treadmill every day isn't likely to be successful, but signing them up for a team sport (like swimming or softball) or lessons (like tennis) might really spark joy in their lives.

TIP

Some question exists about the relationship between strenuous exercise and high blood pressure in children. Find out more about exercise in the nearby sidebar.

>> **Losing weight:** If your child is overweight, you need to help them lose weight by carefully evaluating their current diet and altering it. Suggestions include

- Eliminating obvious sources of empty calories like sodas
- Reducing sources of saturated fat and cholesterol

- Reducing portions of all foods to get the total caloric intake low enough to produce a slow but steady weight loss

REMEMBER

Don't completely deprive your child of the joys of eating. In moderation, a hamburger or pizza can fit into their diet.

>> **Quitting caffeinated beverages:** If your child drinks caffeinated beverages, encourage them to give them up. Energy drinks can contribute to the development of high blood pressure in kids and adolescents.

>> **Quitting smoking and vaping:** Tobacco in any form should be forbidden, whether the child smokes, snuffs, or chews it. A child who has smoked for a fairly brief period will have a much easier time stopping than a child who has had the habit for years. Vaping isn't safe either — the nicotine content in e-cigarettes is significant, and if a child is vaping, they need to quit.

REMEMBER

If you smoke or vape, set an example for your kids by quitting. "Do as I say, not as I do" doesn't really work so well. Head to Chapter 11 for details on kicking the smoking habit.

>> **Quitting illegal drugs:** Illegal drugs like amphetamines and cocaine cause high blood pressure (not to mention being problematic for a variety of other reasons).

>> **Reducing salt consumption:** Salt reduction (see Chapter 10) is key to lowering blood pressure. You can help your child discover how to enjoy the taste of foods that aren't salty. Managing salt intake during childhood may even prevent high blood pressure as an adult.

STRENUOUS EXERCISE IN KIDS WITH HIGH BLOOD PRESSURE

Exercise is important, but if your child's blood pressure is at or greater than the 90th percentile for their age (if they're younger than 13) or over 130/80 mm Hg (if they're 13 or over), talk with their doctor before your child engages in strenuous exercise. Your child may need to start at a lower intensity level and slowly build up to a higher intensity and frequency of exercise over time.

High blood pressure doesn't shut the door to athletic performance, but physical activity must be pursued wisely, especially when the blood pressure is severe or damage to the eyes, kidneys, or heart occurs.

Using Medications

If your child has any of following conditions, they may need to take medication to treat their high blood pressure:

>> Damage to target organs like the heart or kidneys

>> Diabetes

>> Resistant high blood pressure

>> Symptoms such as headaches, nosebleeds, or dizziness

>> Continued high blood pressure despite lifestyle modifications including weight loss, salt reduction, and exercise

The medication treatment for kids with high blood pressure is similar to the treatment of adults (see Chapter 13), though at lower doses:

>> First-line agents in kids include angiotensin-converting enzyme (ACE) inhibitors, angiotensin receptor blockers (ARBs), calcium channel blockers (CCBs), and/or thiazide or thiazide-like diuretics. Just as adults with diabetes do better with ACE inhibitors, kids with diabetes should be given an ACE inhibitor first. Diuretics can be tought for a child to stick with, especially if they have to keep running to the bathroom. CCBs can cause edema in some children; this needs to be watched for when a child first starts taking a CCB.

>> Beta blockers are not the first choice for kids except in specialized situations. The side effects of these medications, especially increased risk of depression and decreased energy levels, make them not the best choice for kids.

TIP

If possible, a single medication taken once a day should be the goal. Kids are often reluctant to take one pill a day, much less two pills two or three times a day.

Frequent monitoring is important prior to starting drug treatment and while a child is taking the drug to monitor the effect of the drug and be sure the child is actually taking the medication. You can do this at home by checking your child's blood pressure regularly.

IN THIS CHAPTER

» **Seeking out salt sensitivity**

» **Finding out about preeclampsia and eclampsia**

» **Taking hormones for contraception and during menopause**

Chapter **17**

Treating High Blood Pressure in Women

igh blood pressure is an important cause of death among women, accounting for approximately 20 percent of all causes of mortality. It can affect women at many different stages of their lives, including before and during pregnancy and after menopause.

Factors that can affect the development of high blood pressure include the use of certain medications (including oral contraceptives), obesity, metabolic syndrome, diabetes, lack of exercise, and increased salt consumption.

This chapter fills you in on all the ways that high blood pressure affects women. You find out how high blood pressure can develop during pregnancy, too, including a discussion on preeclampsia. If you're a woman at risk of developing high blood pressure (or if you've already been diagnosed with high blood pressure), this chapter is for you.

Connecting High Blood Pressure and Salt Sensitivity in Women

When it comes to high blood pressure, women are more sensitive to the effects of sodium intake than men are. Restricting your intake of salt is important for both men and women, but if you're a woman, cutting back on salt will have a big impact!

For women who have gone through menopause, the risk of developing metabolic syndrome (see Chapter 11) increases by more than 50 percent. And high blood pressure associated with metabolic syndrome is due to salt sensitivity. So, reducing salt consumption can really help your blood pressure and improve your overall health. Turn to Chapter 10 for more on reducing your salt intake.

Understanding High Blood Pressure and Pregnancy

During pregnancy, a woman's body goes through many changes to provide the best possible environment for the growing fetus. The mother has to sustain the fetus with nutrition and fluid. To do this, the mother's blood vessels dilate, and the volume of water and salt increases in her blood vessels by an average of more than 40 percent. She gains about 2 gallons of water.

This dilation of blood vessels normally causes the blood pressure to *fall* during the first six months of the pregnancy. (A woman with a history of high blood pressure before pregnancy may even be able to stop high blood pressure medications during pregnancy because her blood pressure may drop into the normal range.)

WARNING

If you're on an angiotensin-converting enzyme (ACE) inhibitor or angiotensin receptor blocker (ARB) and you're planning on becoming pregnant, you'll need to stop the medication for a few months before becoming pregnant because these medications can cause damage to the fetus. Talk with your doctor regarding any medications you're taking if you're planning on becoming pregnant.

TIP

If you have high blood pressure before becoming pregnant, work with your doctor to create a game plan regarding your high blood pressure. Be sure to undergo a complete medical evaluation to evaluate for organ damage related to high blood pressure. (For more on end organ effects of high blood pressure, turn to Part 2.)

HORMONES DURING PREGNANCY

During pregnancy, the increased production of various hormones fosters fetal growth and sustains and prepares your body for delivery and breastfeeding:

- **Estrogen:** An increase in estrogen may be responsible for some of the increased blood flow.

- **Progesterone:** Progesterone increases and helps to maintain the placenta; it also prevents the uterus from contracting.

- **Prolactin:** Prolactin increases during pregnancy in preparation for breastfeeding.

- **Relaxin:** Relaxin, a recently discovered hormone from the placenta, helps to open blood vessels.

- **Renin:** The production of *renin* (an enzyme made by the kidney when it detects a fall in blood pressure) increases during pregnancy. The placenta is also a source of renin.

Knowing what causes high blood pressure during pregnancy

Several factors can cause high blood pressure during pregnancy. Differentiating between high blood pressure that began *before* the pregnancy from high blood pressure that starts *during* the pregnancy is important.

TIP

If you're thinking of becoming pregnant, record your blood pressure. If you develop high blood pressure during pregnancy, you and your doctor will know if your blood pressure developed before or during the pregnancy.

Chronic high blood pressure

Chronic high blood pressure *prior* to pregnancy is recognized as a blood pressure of more than 140/90 mm Hg on repeated occasions, and it's present before pregnancy or recognized before the 20th week of the pregnancy. Because many women haven't had their blood pressure measured before getting pregnant and because blood pressure falls normally during the first six months of pregnancy, chronic high blood pressure may go unnoticed until the final three months of the pregnancy.

Talk with your doctor about your blood pressure. Blood pressure control is very important during pregnancy to maintain the health of both you and your unborn child.

Many blood pressure medications can't be taken during pregnancy. Medications you may be prescribed during pregnancy include methyldopa, labetalol, hydralazine, and/or nifedipine (see Chapter 13).

TIP

A woman who begins a pregnancy with a diagnosis of chronic high blood pressure should be on a modified exercise program under the supervision of a doctor.

WARNING

Chronic high blood pressure poses increased risks to the mother and the fetus. The main risks are as follows:

>> Preeclampsia

>> Problems related to fetal growth

>> Increased risk of fetal mortality

>> Significant worsening of the mother's kidney function if kidney disease is present

Gestational hypertension

Gestational hypertension is high blood pressure usually higher than 140/90 mm Hg that develops after the 20th week of pregnancy but does not include any of the changes that occur with preeclampsia. There is no evidence of any problems with target organs, but mothers with gestational hypertension need to be monitored closely after pregnancy because they're at increased risk of developing high blood pressure. The treatment includes bed rest (hospitalization may be needed if the blood pressure is very elevated), control of blood pressure, and/or delivery of the fetus.

WARNING

If you have gestational hypertension, both you and your fetus will need to be closely monitored during the pregnancy.

Preeclampsia

The traditional definition of preeclampsia was high blood pressure above 140/90 mm Hg with symptoms such as headache, weight gain, blurred vision, swelling, and abdominal pain, along with more than 300 milligrams of protein in the urine in a 24-hour period after the 20th week of pregnancy. The new, expanded definition includes elevated blood pressure with evidence of an organ being affected (such as the liver or kidney), even if there is no protein in the urine.

Preeclampsia is very important to be aware of because, if left unchecked, it can lead to seizures. Treatment is delivery of the baby and placenta.

The risk of preeclampsia is increased if you are having your first baby (especially if you're older than 35) or carrying twins. You're also at higher risk of developing preeclampsia if any of the following apply to you:

>> You had high blood pressure before becoming pregnant.

>> You have diabetes with complications, such as eye disease, kidney disease, or nerve disease.

>> You had any preexisting kidney disease before becoming pregnant.

>> You had preeclampsia in a previous pregnancy.

>> Your mother had preeclampsia.

>> You have a history of systemic lupus erythematosus (SLE).

WARNING

Preeclampsia can have mild, moderate, or severe symptoms. Examples of severe symptoms occur when the blood pressure is 160/110 mm Hg and can include the following:

>> Abdominal pain

>> Abnormal liver enzymes in the blood

>> Blurred vision

>> Excessive and rapid weight gain

>> Headache

>> Low platelet counts in the blood resulting in abnormal clotting and bleeding

>> Increased creatinine level

>> Pulmonary edema

Your doctor will order lab tests if they suspect preeclampsia.

Note: Some pregnant women exhibit certain signs of preeclampsia (headache, nausea, and pain in the abdomen) but don't have high blood pressure. This is known as *HELLP syndrome,* an acronym for *hemolytic anemia, elevated liver enzymes,* and *low platelets,* a serious condition that occurs during the last trimester and sometimes can occur after the delivery of the baby.

Preeclampsia can occur in the postpartum period as well; this is called *postpartum preeclampsia*. If high blood pressure is present or if you're at increased risk for the development of preeclampsia, you'll need to be closely monitored even after giving birth.

One form of treatment that cures preeclampsia is delivery of the baby. When the pregnancy is at 36 weeks or longer, delivery can take place immediately. If the pregnancy hasn't continued to at least the 28th week, however, the fetus may not be mature enough to survive. If the preeclampsia is not worsening and your life is not in danger, the doctor will try to prolong the pregnancy as long as possible. Each extra day means a great deal for the safer delivery of the baby.

Some of the steps the doctor can take to avoid early delivery include

>> **Lowering your blood pressure.** Intravenous medications are often used for an immediate effect.

>> **Giving you magnesium sulfate intravenously to prevent seizures.** Seizures are a complication that turns preeclampsia into eclampsia.

>> **Constantly monitoring both your and the fetus.** Your doctor will monitor your blood pressure, your weight, your urine for protein, and movement of the fetus.

>> **Establishing complete bed rest if the preeclampsia is more severe.**

>> **Continuing a good diet.** To avoid further decreasing your blood volume, you won't reduce your sodium intake.

Given these steps, you and your baby can avoid the complications of preeclampsia, and most mothers can avoid moving from preeclampsia to eclampsia.

After the baby is delivered, your symptoms will usually disappear in a few days or weeks unless the injury to certain organs is severe.

Dealing with eclampsia

If you're diagnosed with preeclampsia and you develop seizures, the condition is called *eclampsia*. Fortunately, eclampsia occurs rarely — in about 3 percent of pregnancies in the United States — but it can threaten the life of the mother and the fetus.

Eclampsia results from severe narrowing of the blood vessels in the brain of the mother, which then diminishes the supply of nutrients to the brain cells. Seizures usually take place before the baby is delivered, but they can occur after delivery, too. High blood pressure may not always be present, but usually it is.

PREECLAMPSIA ON TOP OF CHRONIC HIGH BLOOD PRESSURE

When preeclampsia complicates chronic high blood pressure during a pregnancy, the risks for the mother and the fetus are greater than the risks from either condition alone. Determining whether the chronic high blood pressure is getting worse or preeclampsia is beginning may be difficult, but a number of signs point to the onset of preeclampsia. The most useful of these signs are

- Protein in the urine when previous tests showed none

- A sudden increase in protein in the urine

- A sudden increase in high blood pressure that has previously been controlled

- A platelet count in the blood of less than 100,000 per cubic millimeter, which means a tendency to bleed easily

- Abnormal liver function

The treatment of preeclampsia in association with chronic high blood pressure is even more urgent than the treatment of preeclampsia alone. The decision to end such a pregnancy is made even earlier than when high blood pressure isn't a complication.

To treat eclampsia, your doctor will administer magnesium sulfate to stop the convulsions. If necessary, your blood pressure will be controlled with medication into the vein. The fetus will undergo continuous monitoring.

When everything appears to be more stable (usually within hours), the doctor delivers the baby. Although vaginal delivery is preferable, a Cesarean section is performed if time is critical.

After delivery, you'll have to continue to take magnesium sulfate for several days until the signs of preeclampsia and eclampsia are clearly diminishing.

Dealing with high blood pressure after delivery

If you have chronic high blood pressure, you can take a few medications to help manage your high blood pressure while you're breastfeeding. These medications include methyldopa, hydralazine, labetalol, and nifedipine. Turn to Chapter 13 for more on these medications.

If you're breastfeeding, ask your doctor about *all* medications you're taking, not just medications for blood pressure.

Using Hormone Treatments If You Have High Blood Pressure

Women take estrogen and progesterone for two major indications: to prevent pregnancy and to replace missing hormones after menopause. Although earlier formulations were associated with increases in blood pressure, the current treatments are only occasionally associated with an increase in blood pressure. The following sections guide you through hormone use that avoids triggering high blood pressure.

Oral contraceptives

Just exactly how oral contraceptives raise blood pressure is unknown. No particular factor (like weight, age, or ethnic origin) seems to predict who will have an increase in blood pressure and to what extent. In the past, most women who took oral contraceptives had a rise in blood pressure that was usually mild, but rarely severe. Newer oral contraceptives contain much smaller doses of both estrogen and progesterone. Today, the increase in blood pressure is less frequent, probably as a result of the reduced dosage. That being said, oral contraceptives can still raise blood pressure, so your blood pressure needs to be monitored if you start taking one.

Women who smoke and are over age 35 are more sensitive to oral contraceptives and shouldn't take them. The combination of oral contraceptives and smoking also increases the risk of developing blood clots in the legs and the lungs. Although the rise in blood pressure doesn't cause damage for most of these women, occasionally the kidneys are damaged. If your doctor is concerned about your blood pressure, you should discontinue the oral contraceptive, which will cause a prompt fall in your blood pressure.

If you plan to take oral contraceptives, stop smoking (a good idea even if you don't plan to take them!). Make sure your blood pressure is measured before you start the contraceptive and every six months while you take it. If you have a blood pressure increase of 20 mm Hg systolic or 10 mm Hg diastolic, replace the oral contraceptive with a different form of contraception.

Hormone replacement therapy

After menopause, high blood pressure can increase, so any medication that can turn that condition into high blood pressure must be carefully evaluated. Hormone replacement therapy (HRT) uses estrogen, though in much lower doses than oral contraceptives do. A form of estrogen that has been useful in lowering blood pressure is *transdermal estrogen* (estrogen given as a patch or gel applied to the skin). Other formulations with progestin may also help with lowering blood pressure.

REMEMBER

HRT can have risks and benefits. If HRT is started before the age of 60, for example, there is a reduction in the risk of heart disease but an increased stroke risk. HRT needs to be personalized. The bottom line: Talk with your doctor before starting HRT. They know your individual health history and can discuss the risks and benefits of HRT with you.

5

The Part of Tens

Chapter **18**

Ten Simple Ways to Prevent or Reduce High Blood Pressure

In this chapter, you read about ten possible ways to prevent or lower high blood pressure. Many of them are easy to incorporate into your daily life — from adjusting your nutrition plan to adding a touch of meditation to reducing or even eliminating smoking. Your initial goal should be to adopt one or two of these ideas. After that, try adding an additional one each month. Each idea you're able to adopt will improve your overall health and well-being. Any action that you take is better than nothing at all — this isn't all or nothing. When is the best time to make changes in your health and well-being? Today, now, as soon as you've finished reading this chapter! In the immortal words of Shakespeare in *Henry VI, Part 3*, "Strike now, or else the iron cools."

Know Your Blood Pressure

You may save yourself a lifetime of taking unnecessary blood pressure medication by simply making sure your blood pressure is *truly* elevated, so the first step is to be certain it's *persistently* elevated.

Make sure your health-care provider is measuring your blood pressure properly (see Chapter 2) because numerous aspects can affect the accuracy:

>> The size of the blood pressure cuff

>> The placement of the cuff on your arm

>> Whether you're relaxed before the measurement

>> Whether you're quiet (not speaking) during the measurement

In addition, make sure you don't have *white-coat high blood pressure* (blood pressure that's high only in the doctor's office when you may be anxious). A good home blood pressure device properly calibrated can check for this possibility. (See Chapter 2 for an entire section on home monitoring.)

WARNING

Don't rely on readings obtained from pharmacy measurement devices — they have a high error rate.

Know Whether You Have Resistant High Blood Pressure

About 5 percent of high blood pressure cases are difficult to control with medication, which means the diagnosis is *resistant high blood pressure.* If your health-care provider can discover the cause and treat the underlying condition, especially early on, it may help to eliminate your high blood pressure (and possibly the need for medication) and perhaps prevent other damage to your body.

REMEMBER

Resistant high blood pressure may be present if any of the following apply to you:

>> You have high blood pressure that develops suddenly and you're under the age of 18 or over the age of 50.

>> You're resistant to four or more blood pressure medications (or three medications if one of the medications is a diuretic).

>> You've had changes in body shape and/or pigmentation.

>> You've had episodes of fast heart rate, dizziness, coldness, and/or paleness, along with high blood pressure.

>> You have no family history of high blood pressure.

TECHNICAL STUFF

If your health-care provider suspects resistant high blood pressure, they should test for at least primary hyperaldosteronism, which is undiagnosed and likely responsible for more than 25 percent of undiagnosed resistant high blood pressure. (See Chapter 4 for the nuances on diagnosing this important condition.) Kidney function also should be checked to evaluate for chronic kidney disease, the most common cause of resistant high blood pressure.

Adopt the DASH Diet

In 1997, a study published in the *New England Journal of Medicine* introduced the Dietary Approach to Stop Hypertension (DASH) diet. This diet (see Chapter 9) may have been the best treatment for high blood pressure in decades.

The DASH diet requires you to eat a mix of grains, fruits, and vegetables and low-fat or nonfat dairy products while you reduce your intake of high-fat dairy products, meats, fats, and sweets. The diet also encourages a weekly amount of nuts and seeds.

TIP

You don't have to change your diet all at once, but it is important to start making changes. Start by reducing your intake of meat and dairy and substitute some grains. Add more vegetables. Have fruit for dessert instead of cookies, cake, or ice cream. Before you know it, you'll be "DASHing"!

Combining DASH (where salt reduction takes place automatically) with even further reduction in sodium can double the effects of lowering your high blood pressure. Don't add salt to food, and try to keep your sodium intake under 1,500 milligrams per day.

TIP

After you read Chapter 9, consider the services of a knowledgeable nutritionist. Make sure they're well versed in the requirements of DASH and elements of plant-based nutrition.

Cut Out the Caffeine

Don't underestimate the effect caffeine can have on your blood pressure (see Chapter 10). A great way to lower your blood pressure is by reducing the amount of caffeine you consume. Decrease the amount of coffee you're drinking by half or consider consuming a "half-caf" drink with half regular coffee and half decaffeinated if you still need a little bit of a morning jolt to get you going in the morning. Decreasing you caffeine intake can do a lot to help improve your blood pressure.

REMEMBER

Don't forget other sources of caffeine that you may consume on a daily basis and not think about, including tea, soda, energy drinks, and some over-the-counter supplements or herbs.

Reduce the Amount of Salt in Your Diet

One of the easiest ways to bring down your blood pressure is to decrease your intake of sodium. Don't worry that you won't get enough — you need only 500 milligrams of sodium a day, which you can get if you eat only natural foods. Most Americans consume 5,000 milligrams per day, so 1,500 milligrams is a more realistic goal.

TIP

Prepared foods account for 75 percent of the salt in the average American's diet, so consider these suggestions:

>> Cut back on the number of prepared foods you buy (for example, prepared soups and crackers).

>> Consult the Nutrition Facts label on each item to check the amount of sodium in each portion. Even if the sodium content appears low, eating too many portions can put your sodium level over the top.

>> Cut back on chips and crackers.

Substitute low-salt chips or, even better, fresh fruits or raw vegetables for snacks high in salt.

Another 10 percent of the salt that you eat occurs naturally in food, but the final 15 percent is from the saltshaker. Try keeping the saltshaker off the table — out of sight, out of mind. After a few days, you'll be surprised how much food tastes when it isn't blunted by salt.

TIP

If you still need additional flavor, try adding herbs and spices. If you're using canned vegetables, try washing out most of the salt with plain water and then add herbs and spices.

Monitoring the amount of salt in your food is difficult when you eat out. Chefs tend to add salt liberally. But you can ask for the food to be prepared with little or no salt or choose a restaurant that offers low-sodium items on the menu. Plan ahead and look at the menu ahead of time before going out. You can have an enjoyable dinner and eat healthy at the same time!

Give Up Tobacco and Alcohol

Both tobacco and alcohol can raise blood pressure (see Chapter 11). Consider these facts:

REMEMBER

>> **Because of the nicotine content, tobacco in any form (smoked, chewed, or snuffed) raises blood pressure through a couple of different mechanisms.** About one-third of people with high blood pressure are smokers. Plus, smoking accelerates atherosclerosis and tremendously increases the risk of heart disease and peripheral vascular disease.

Any regular exposure to tobacco is dangerous. If you smoke, you're damaging your own health *and* compromising the health of your loved ones through the effects of secondhand smoke. Spouses and children of smokers have a much higher rate of lung disease, asthma, and cancer than the spouses and children of nonsmokers. When you stop smoking, you and everyone around you benefits.

>> **Consuming excess alcohol can raise blood pressure.** Even a daily alcoholic beverage can be harmful to your liver and is not recommended.

Start an Exercise Program

Choose an exercise program that you enjoy and can adhere to. Just like a sound nutritional plan, an exercise plan will not only treat but also prevent the development of high blood pressure.

REMEMBER

Make sure you're healthy enough to begin an exercise program by visiting your health-care provider.

TIP

Something as fundamental as regularly walking is a good initial step and works very well for many people (see Chapter 12 for a complete program and its benefits). Design your program to start slowly for short distances and build up over time to 45 minutes of exercise three or four times a week.

Don't forget the benefits of muscle resistance training in addition to aerobic exercise (like walking). Again, talk with your health-care provider first to see if you're healthy enough to handle resistance training. Then call a gym associated with your local hospital or health system and talk to a licensed exercise physiologist to do some additional testing and get a personalized treatment plan. This approach will reduce your risk of injury.

REMEMBER

Exercise doesn't just lower blood pressure — it improves self-esteem, improves balance, fights depression, enhances memory, and generally makes you very aware that life is worth living!

Practice Mind-Body Techniques

The incorporation of, mind-body techniques such as yoga and meditation can enhance your well-being and lower your blood pressure. If you can lower your blood pressure just a little, and reap other benefits at the same time (like a more focused and serene mind), it's worthwhile. (See Chapter 12 for more information on mind-body techniques.)

REMEMBER

Examples of mind-body techniques include the following:

>> **Yoga:** Yoga emphasizes postures and proper breathing. Individuals who finished a yoga class almost always express how relaxed and warm they feel. When their blood pressure is taken, it's often lower than before the class started.

>> **Meditation:** Meditation calms the mind by concentrating on an object, a sound, a word, or the breath. Just a few minutes once or twice a day to start may be enough to help control your blood pressure.

>> **Deep breathing:** Meditation includes controlled, deep breathing, but deep breathing does not necessary include meditation. By controlling your breathing (see Chapter 12), you can help lower your blood pressure by reducing/decreasing the intensity of your body's fight-or-flight response.

>> **Biofeedback:** This technique uses a *biofeedback machine* to detect a person's internal bodily functions (such as high blood pressure) in order to alter a function. Because biofeedback requires equipment, it may be a little less desirable than the other methods. But if you can't engage in the other mind-body techniques, this may be the solution for you.

TIP

Deep breathing can be an effective way of combating white-coat high blood pressure, especially when you're about to have your blood pressure taken in a doctor's office.

Take Your Medication

The prescribing of a medication (not only for blood pressure but for any medical condition) should, in my opinion, be a shared decision between a patient and their health-care provider. It involves an open and honest discussion of the proposed medication to be prescribed, including its benefits, possible side effects, and possible adverse reactions.

Understanding how each medication you're taking works is especially important because some blood pressure medications (such as beta blockers and clonidine) can't be stopped cold turkey. (Doing so can induce a withdrawal reaction, causing very high blood pressure and a rapid heart rate.) Medications like these need to be gradually decreased if you want or need to stop.

REMEMBER

Don't hesitate to call your health-care provider if you have a concern regarding your blood pressure medication. Lowering your blood pressure is a team effort.

Avoid Medications That Raise Blood Pressure

Some medications that are prescribed can antagonize or block the action of a blood pressure medication, whether this medication is prescribed or available over the counter. For example, not only can nonsteroidal anti-inflammatories (NSAIDs) raise blood pressure due to sodium and water retention, but they can also block the blood-pressure-lowering actions of a class of medications called diuretics (see Chapter 13).

TIP

Keep an updated medication list with you at all times, including any medications, supplements, and herbal medications that you take. Check your electronic health record (EHR) and make sure the medications listed are correct.

REMEMBER

Some medications may raise blood pressure in only one person — you! Why? Because we're all different, and medications can react differently in each of us. It's important that allergies and adverse reactions (and the nature of those reactions) are included in your medication record as well.

Check with your health-care provider and monitor your blood pressure whenever you start or stop a new medication.

REMEMBER

Cold medications may contain ingredients like ephedrine or pseudoephedrine that constrict arteries and elevate blood pressure. Read the labels on any cold medication that you plan to use. Any medication that can affect blood pressure has a label clearly stating that it should *not* be taken by a person who has high blood pressure. If you're not sure if a medication is safe to take, check with your health-care provider or ask the pharmacist.

Prescription medications that may raise blood pressure include the following:

» Steroids like cortisone or prednisone

» Several antidepressant medications

- Trimipramine and venlafaxine in particular cause sustained increases in blood pressure.

- Antidepressant drugs from the monoamine oxidase inhibitors class raise blood pressure by preventing the breakdown of epinephrine. Drugs in this class include phenelzine and tranylcypromine.

» NSAIDs, including ibuprofen (brand name: Advil), indomethacin (brand name: Tivorbex), and naproxen (brand name: Aleve)

Oral contraceptives used to contain high amounts of estrogen, which made them notorious for raising blood pressure. The newer preparations with less estrogen are much better, but your blood pressure should be checked before you start and monitored while you're on them.

Antacids can contain an abundance of salt that can affect your blood pressure. Check the label! Other options include calcium- and magnesium-containing antacids.

Illegal drugs such as cocaine and methamphetamine raise blood pressure and obviously shouldn't be taken in the first place.

Chapter **19**

Ten (or So) Myths about High Blood Pressure

Despite how common high blood pressure is, many myths persist about it, some of which I debunk in this chapter. Read on to find out the truth about this preventable and treatable condition.

High Blood Pressure Is Inevitable as You Get Older

High blood pressure is *not* an inevitable part of aging. It's a result of a poor diet (deficient in fruits and vegetables, with too much sodium) and too little exercise. One of the risk factors for high blood pressure *is* age, but poor diet and lack of exercise can cause high blood pressure even in younger people. And in plenty of populations in rural areas in different parts of the world, high blood pressure is nonexistent or rare, even among older people.

Approximately 30 percent of older people in the United States do *not* have high blood pressure. However, people who *do* have high blood pressure tend to have several other factors in common:

>> Increased body mass index (BMI). (To find your BMI, search the web for "BMI calculator" or go to www.nhlbi.nih.gov/health/educational/lose_wt/BMI/bmicalc.htm.)

>> Being out of shape.

>> A processed diet (not plant based).

>> A diet high in sodium and/or sugar.

The one change that occurs with age that may lead to high blood pressure is a gradual loss of kidney function with the development of chronic kidney disease. However, this loss may be related to the factors in the previous list rather than to aging itself.

REMEMBER

You *can* prevent high blood pressure by adopting a healthy lifestyle at a young age and sticking to it. The result is not just a longer life but also a higher-quality life. Turn to Part 3 for the lifestyle changes you can make to prevent (or reduce) high blood pressure.

The Treatment Is Worse Than the Disease

The consequences of untreated high blood pressure at *any* age are far greater than the side effects of medication or the inconveniences of lifestyle changes. For example, when you use non-pharmacologic treatments — like lowering your sodium and caffeine intake and exercising regularly — your blood pressure responds. (Turn to Chapters 8 through 12 for more ways that you can adjust your lifestyle to lower your blood pressure.)

REMEMBER

Many non-pharmacologic treatments provide all kinds of other benefits. The inner peace and serenity that comes from exercising, doing yoga, and meditating can't be found in any in any blood pressure medication.

After you speak with your health-care provider, if you need blood pressure medication, it pays to take it. The consequences of uncontrolled blood pressure — heart attack, stroke, and/or kidney disease — are far worse than the side effects of any blood pressure medication.

If you do experience side effects from blood pressure medication, you can deal with them in several ways:

>> **Ask your doctor whether you can lower your dose while monitoring your blood pressure.** Don't lower your dose on your own — talk with your doctor first.

>> **If side effects are severe, ask your doctor if they can prescribe two different medications at lower doses.** This may help you to avoid the side effects of either one.

Certain drugs called *angiotensin-converting enzyme inhibitors* are especially helpful under special circumstances like diabetic kidney disease, but they cause side effects. Instead of losing the great benefits of these drugs, ask your doctor whether you can switch. For example, if cough is your problem, switch to an angiotensin II receptor blocker.

>> **If you're fatigued, ask your doctor to check your potassium level and do other blood work, as well as considering adjusting your blood pressure medications.**

>> **If you perform some work that requires high mental alertness (like running heavy equipment or driving a car), let your health-care provider know.** Work with your doctor to determine the combination of lifestyle changes and medications that are right for you.

You Must Restrict Your Life Because You Have High Blood Pressure

Although high blood pressure is a serious condition that has to be managed with lifestyle changes and sometimes medication, restricting your life (for example, by avoiding strenuous exercise or never eating out) isn't reasonable. The side effects of blood pressure drugs shouldn't keep you from living the life you want to live.

If you have to adjust your diet to a plant-based one, try not to think about it as restricting your diet. Instead, think of it as enhancing the quality of your life. You have a chance to taste some *amazing* foods that were hidden behind the strong taste of salt. Plus, you'll feel better and be healthier! Sometimes just a shift in attitude is all it takes to make changing a little easier.

You Only Need Treatment If You Have High Systolic Blood Pressure

In medical school, some doctors were trained to focus on lowering the systolic blood pressure (the top number), and you may have heard this same thing somewhere along the way. Systolic blood pressure is important, but it isn't the only number you have to pay attention to.

REMEMBER

Both the diastolic blood pressure (the lower number) and the systolic blood pressure are important (see Chapter 2 for more information about these two numbers).

TECHNICAL STUFF

Diastolic blood pressure tends to fall with age, whereas systolic blood pressure tends to rise. Treating high blood pressure is important, but lowering the diastolic blood pressure *too* much in older people is dangerous. If it drops below around 65 mmHg to 70 mmHg with blood pressure medication, a person is actually at increased risk of stroke. In these cases, you may have to accept a systolic blood pressure greater than 140 in order to avoid a diastolic blood pressure below 70. Your doctor will monitor your blood pressure and your body's response to medication and find the medication and dosage that's right for you.

If You Have High Blood Pressure, You'll Have to Take Medication Forever

All you have to do is read Part 3 of this book to see that having high blood pressure does *not* mean you have to take medication for the rest of your life.

REMEMBER

Medications are used when lifestyle changes are not enough to lower your blood pressure. But even then, by changing your lifestyle, your doctor may be able to decrease the dosage of the medication(s) that you're taking. When you lower your blood pressure by a *little* bit, you reduce the risk of stroke, heart attack, and kidney and eye damage.

You Can Stop Treatment after a Heart Attack or Stroke

If you've had a heart attack or stroke, keeping your blood pressure under control is more important than ever! One of the main risk factors for a heart attack or stroke is a *previous* heart attack or stroke. So, after you recover, you *must* continue your treatment. Before you leave the hospital, plan to make the changes that can bring your blood pressure under control:

>> Stop smoking.

>> Reduce or completely eliminate your consumption of alcohol.

>> Follow a low-salt, plant-based diet.

>> Start a lifelong exercise program (after your doctor has given you the green light to do so).

Turn to Part 3 for more information on all these lifestyle changes.

REMEMBER

The changes that you adopt to help you control your high blood pressure can also help with diabetes, arthritis, and more.

You Should Avoid Exercise If You Have High Blood Pressure

Many people who have high blood pressure and don't want to exercise fall back on this myth. The problem is, it's completely false. Exercise *lowers* blood pressure. Even just 30 minutes of walking a day provides great benefits! The key is to find a form of exercise that you enjoy — that way, you'll be more likely to stick with it!

REMEMBER

If you have heart disease or you've had a heart attack or stroke, ask your health-care provider what exercises you can do safely. You may have no limitations, or you may need to avoid activities that are too vigorous or require too much effort over a short period of time (like heavy weightlifting). Depending on your health history and the exercise regimen you're thinking about embarking upon, you may need to talk with an exercise physiologist.

Many health-care systems have gyms and trained personnel who can assess your capabilities and create a personalized exercise program for you (see Chapter 12).

If You're Feeling Good, You Can Stop Taking Your Blood Pressure Meds

High blood pressure is called the "silent killer" because people are often unaware they have it. The disease can even damage the eyes, heart, kidneys, and blood vessels before symptoms appear — and then it's often too late to reverse the damage.

REMEMBER

Take your blood pressure medication! The point is to lower your blood pressure so you can prevent complications like heart attack and stroke in the future. These complications can take years to develop, so the sooner you bring your blood pressure down into the normal range, the more time you have to avoid these risks.

TIP

If side effects from the medication are a problem, talk to your doctor about the possibility of lowering the dose or switching to another medicine.

High Blood Pressure Can't Be Controlled

If you take your medication regularly but your blood pressure doesn't come down into the acceptable range, don't give up — and definitely don't stop taking your medication! Instead, with the help of your health-care provider, review your current medication regimen, diet, and lifestyle to see what else you can do to control your blood pressure.

Rest assured, there is often an explanation and a way to control your high blood pressure. As a team, you and your health-care provider can find the right solution. Here are some questions to talk about with your health-care provider:

>> **Are you sure my blood pressure is uncontrolled?** Could it be a faulty measurement? Is your blood pressure normal except when you step into the doctor's office (this is called the *white-coat effect;* see Chapter 2)? What is your blood pressure doing at home?

>> **Is another medication I'm taking interfering with my high blood pressure medication?** Make sure your doctor is aware of all the medications you take.

>> **Have I changed my lifestyle enough?** Are you reducing your salt and sugar intake? Have you tried a plant-based diet? Have you quit smoking? Have you reduced or eliminated your intake of caffeine? Have you tried yoga, meditation, or other stress reduction techniques?

TIP

Discuss with your health care provider the possibility that you have resistant high blood pressure (see Chapter 4). The diseases and conditions that can cause resistant high blood pressure (blocked kidney arteries or a tumor in an adrenal gland, for example) are rare but may account for the stubborn resistance of your blood pressure to treatment.

People with High Blood Pressure Are Just Nervous or Anxious

A high level of nervousness and anxiety is not an indication that a person has or will have high blood pressure. In fact, a nervous, anxious person may have normal blood pressure, and a person who appears quite calm and peaceful may have exceedingly high blood pressure.

This myth probably developed from the technical name for high blood pressure — *hypertension*. The prefix *hyper* suggests that sufferers are highly stressed, jumpy, and nervous people who live a life of anger and road rage and have a short fuse that's ready to blow at any moment. The suffix *tension* certainly doesn't suggest a calm, peaceful state of being.

REMEMBER

Individuals with high blood pressure are everywhere doing every type of work. Stress is a risk factor, but stress is usually not the only cause for persistent high blood pressure.

Older People Don't Need to Be Treated

People over the age of 65 are more likely to have high blood pressure and suffer heart attacks and strokes. Despite this fact, the myth persists that if you're older, it's too late or not helpful to treat high blood pressure. But treating older people for high blood pressure can prevent major events like heart attack and stroke.

High Blood Pressure Is Less Dangerous in Women

The consequences of high blood pressure for women are just as serious as they are for men, so controlling it is just as important for women (see Chapter 17).

There are many women with uncontrolled high blood pressure, and high blood pressure affects women of all ages.

WARNING

As a result of high blood pressure, *preeclampsia* and *eclampsia* are two extremely dangerous disorders that can begin in the 20th week of pregnancy. These conditions are serious — they increase the risk of death for both the mother and the baby.

TIP

Estrogen may play an important role in women who are postmenopausal with high blood pressure. Estrogen replacement therapy can lower blood pressure.

Appendix

Resources

A wealth of information about high blood pressure is waiting for you from respected and trusted organizations and publications. In this appendix, I steer you toward resources you can trust.

National Heart, Lung, and Blood Institute

The National Heart, Lung, and Blood Institute's website (www.nhlbi.nih.gov) is a great resource for understanding more about high blood pressure. (You can also call them at 877-645-2448 or write to NHLBI Center for Health Information, P.O. Box 30105, Bethesda, MD 20824.) In 1972, the institute began creating public education programs to assist in the reduction of high blood pressure and its complications.

The website also many resources concerning high blood pressure. As of this writing, on the index page (www.nhlbi.nih.gov/health), you can find many topics to search, depending on your area of interest. Besides the basic information, the website includes tips and quizzes, information about medications and working with your doctor, and real-life examples of people with high blood pressure.

If you want more information, go to www.nhlbi.nih.gov/contact and follow the links for an answer to just about any question on high blood pressure.

TIP

For information on the National High Blood Pressure Education Month (each May), check out www.nhlbi.nih.gov/education/high-blood-pressure/high-blood-pressure-education-month.

National Kidney Foundation

The kidneys are organs that may contribute to high blood pressure and also be affected by it (see Chapter 6). The National Kidney Foundation's website (www.kidney.org) has important information on the kidneys in general and specific help regarding high blood pressure and the kidneys. The website also has information on donor family support, nutrition, treatment, rehabilitation, organ donation, and health-care services.

National Institute of Diabetes and Digestive and Kidney Diseases

The National Institute of Diabetes and Digestive and Kidney Diseases website (www.niddk.nih.gov) has valuable information on all aspects of diabetes, gastrointestinal disease, and kidney disease. This is important because diabetes and high blood pressure often occur together. You can access information specific to high blood pressure and the kidneys at www.niddk.nih.gov/health-information/kidney-disease. This area of the site provides answers for how high blood pressure damages the kidneys, how you can prevent it, and what to do if kidney damage has already occurred. (See Chapter 6 for more information about the effect of high blood pressure on the kidneys.)

TIP

The website also links to numerous publications on all aspects of kidney disease (for example, you can find extensive descriptions of dialysis techniques).

American Heart and Stroke Associations

The American Stroke Association (www.stroke.org) is a division of the American Heart Association (www.heart.org). Both associations' websites offer extensive information for professionals and patients, providing thousands of pages of information and links to other resources on high blood pressure and stroke (see Chapter 7 for more on strokes).

The American Heart Association's mission is to reduce complications from cardiovascular disease and stroke. The website is a great source of information about high blood pressure, as well as heart disease.

The American Stroke Association site offers information about the prevention of stroke (see Chapter 7), caring for someone who has had a stroke, medical resources, and just about anything you need to know for dealing with this complication of high blood pressure. The website provides links to the most common symptoms, recovery and rehabilitation, stroke risk, a description of a stroke, acute treatment, and the effects of stroke on affected individuals and their families.

National Library of Medicine

The U.S. National Library of Medicine website (www.nlm.nih.gov) provides links to MedlinePlus and PubMed (see the following sections).

MedlinePlus

MedlinePlus (https://medlineplus.gov) has hundreds of discussions of health topics from the National Institutes of Health. Go to https://medlineplus.gov/highbloodpressure.html for discussions specific to high blood pressure. You can find information on everything from the diagnosis and treatment of high blood pressure to important nutrition information to blood pressure monitoring and more.

MedlinePlus also provides

>> A medical encyclopedia and dictionaries

>> Extensive information on prescription and nonprescription drugs

>> Health information from newspaper and magazine sources

>> Health information in Spanish

>> Links to thousands of clinical trials

>> Lists of hospitals and physicians by state

Like all government websites, MedlinePlus doesn't carry any advertisements or endorsements.

TIP

If you have an email address, you can sign up for MedlinePlus weekly updates.

PubMed

You can search PubMed (www.pubmed.gov) for any medical term. In this case, type in **high blood pressure** and click Search to see thousands of references. If you want to limit your search to certain types of literature (such as reviews of a particular subject within a certain time span), you can filter your search.

The fact that you can access thousands of articles on any medical topic online is amazing. If you need justification for paying your federal taxes, the PubMed website serves that function well. Did I just write "justification for paying your federal taxes"? Oh, well.

The Mayo Clinic

The world-renowned Mayo Clinic has a website (www.mayoclinic.org) with extensive material on every aspect of disease, including high blood pressure. Going to the Mayo Clinic website is like sitting down with a super-easy-to-understand medical textbook. When you click Health Library and then Diseases & Conditions (or just go straight to www.mayoclinic.org/diseases-conditions), you can find links to various other pages, links to other useful websites, and discussions on high blood pressure.

American College of Lifestyle Medicine

As you know from reading this book, lifestyle modifications are very important not only for blood pressure control but for overall health. Did you know that there is a specialty in medicine called "lifestyle medicine"? There are health-care providers who have specialized training in this area. If you're looking for a health-care professional with this specialized training, go to the website of the American College of Lifestyle Medicine (https://lifestylemedicine.org/patient) and click Find a Clinician (or just go straight to www.lifestylemedpros.org). The American College of Lifestyle Medicine website also has a lot of good information on important lifestyle choices, such as plant-based medicine (which is excellent for your blood pressure!).

Centers for Disease Control and Prevention

The Centers for Disease Control and Prevention (CDC) is a great resource on high blood pressure. The website has a whole section on high blood pressure (www.cdc.gov/bloodpressure), including featured resources to learn more about risk factors and prevention.

Index

Numbers

1 alpha hydroxylase D, 73

A

abdominal exam, 21

abdominal swelling, 63

ACCORD (Action to Control Cardiovascular Risk in Diabetes), 188–189

accurate blood pressure readings, 15–17, 223–224

ACE (angiotensin-converting enzyme) inhibitors, 35, 65, 163–167, 212

ACTH (adrenocorticotrophin), 43–44

Action in Diabetes and Vascular Disease (ADVANCE), 189

acute thrombotic stroke, 88

Addiction & Recovery For Dummies (Ritvo), 137

adenomas, 36

adrenal cortex, 39–40

adrenal glands, 36

adrenaline, 130

adrenocorticotrophin (ACTH), 43–44

ADVANCE (Action in Diabetes and Vascular Disease), 189

aerobic activities, 144, 147

African-Americans, 25–26, 108

age of onset, 31

Agency for Healthcare Research and Quality, 136

AHA/ACC (American Heart Association/American College of Cardiology), 18

alcohol, 20, 27

  consequences of drinking, 227

  linking to high blood pressure, 136–137

  tyramine in, 38

aldosterone, 72

  defined, 36

  hyperaldosteronism, 39–43

aldosterone-antagonist diuretics, 161–162

aldosterone-producing adenoma, 42

alpha-1 adrenergic receptor antagonists, 174–175

ambulatory blood pressure monitoring, 15, 17

America diet, 110

American Cancer Society, 136

American Heart Association/American College of Cardiology (AHA/ACC), 18

American Journal of Cardiology, 151

American Journal of Hypertension, 151

American Journal of Medicine, 122

American Lung Association, 136

American Medical Association, 17

amiloride, 161

amlodipine, 169

anaerobic exercises, 144

anemia, 137

aneroid blood pressure gauge, 14

aneurysms, 90, 97, 103

angina, 57–58

anginal equivalents, 57

angioneurotic edema, 164

angioplasty, 34–35, 61

angiotensin II receptor blockers (ARBs), 42, 167–168, 212

angiotensin-converting enzyme (ACE) inhibitors, 35, 65, 163–167, 212

annual health assessment, 9

antacids, 230

anti-anxiety medications, 20

anticoagulants, 60, 93

antidepressants, 20, 26, 230

anti-inflammatory drugs, 156

antiplatelet drugs, 93

anxiety, 237

aorta

  coarctation of, 46

  providing blood flow, 32, 52

aortic valve, 19

apoplexy, 88

ARAS (atherosclerotic renal artery stenosis), 33

ARBs (angiotensin II receptor blockers), 42, 167–168, 212

Archives of General Medicine, 122

arms
  blood pressure in, 16
  weakness in, 94
arrhythmias, 93
arteries, 8, 54, 196
arteriosclerosis, 53, 55–56, 103
arthritis, 197, 201
aspirin, 93
Association for Applied Psychophysiology and
    Biofeedback, 152
asthma, 172
atenolol, 172
atherosclerosis, 88–89
atherosclerotic plaque, 66, 90
atherosclerotic renal artery stenosis (ARAS), 33
atria, 52
atrial fibrillation, 90, 93
automated blood pressure gauge, 187
  buying, 17
  overview, 14
autonomic neuropathy, 202

B

balloon angioplasty, 46
baseline high blood pressure, 195
basketball, 148
bed rest, 216
benazepril, 165
beta blockers (beta-adrenergic receptor blockers), 60, 65,
    171–174
biking, 147, 148
bilateral adrenal hyperplasia, 42
biofeedback, 151–152, 228
birth defects, 139
bisoprolol, 173
bladder, 70
bladder, sphygmomanometer, 14
bladder cancer, 131
blood
  blocking flow to heart muscle, 53–54
  in cardiovascular system, 8, 19
  going through kidneys, 71
blood pressure
  in children, 205–206
  measuring, 8–9, 15–17

in older people, 195–197
  considering resistant high blood pressure, 196–197
  examining medications, 197
  recognizing baseline high blood pressure, 195
blood urea nitrogen (BUN) level, 74
body fat distribution, 21
body mass index (BMI), 115–117
bone density, 131
brain hemorrhage, 90–91
brain imaging, 95–97
brand names, medications, 182–184
breast lumps, 139
breastfeeding, 156
  ACE inhibitors during, 164
  angiotensin II receptor blockers, 167
  methyldopa, 170
  nifedipine, 169
bruit, 31, 33
bumetanide, 160
BUN (blood urea nitrogen) level, 74
bupropion SR, 135–136
bypass surgery, 61

C

CABG (coronary artery bypass grafting), 61
caffeine, 137–140
  children drinking, 209
  cutting out, 225–226
  daily recommended maximum amount of, 138
  health consequences of, 139
  reducing intake of, 139–140
calcium, 56, 109
calcium channel blockers (CCBs), 60, 168–170
Calm app, 151
calories
  burned during exercises, 148
  determining daily caloric needs, 116–118
candesartan, 167
canned foods, 126
capillaries, 8
captopril, 165–166
carbohydrates, 127
cardiac enzymes (troponin levels), 58
cardiovascular disease, 15
cardiovascular system, 8, 52–53

carvedilol, 174

Caucasians, 26, 108

CBC (complete blood count), 22

CCBs (calcium channel blockers), 60, 168–170

CDC (Centers for Disease Control and Prevention), 136
  cigarettes smoked in US, 130
  heart attack mortality rate, 56
  prevalence of high blood pressure
    among different ethnicities, 25–26
    in children, 203
    in US, 1, 7
  secondhand smoke deaths, 132
  stroke prevalence, 87

cerebral embolus, 89–90

cerebrovascular accident, 88

chambers of the heart, 53

cheat sheet, for this book, 3

check ups, before starting exercise, 143

cheeses, tyramine in, 38

chemotherapy medications, 26

chewing tobacco, 132

children, 203–210
  causes of elevated blood pressure in, 206–207
    hereditary influences, 206–207
    weight, 207
  coarctation of the aorta, 46
  evaluating in, 11
  FMD in, 33
  lifestyle changes, 208–209
  measuring blood pressure, 204–206
    interpreting results, 205–206
    on tiny arms, 204–205
  using medications, 210

chlorthalidone, 157

chocolate, 139

cholesterol, 66, 92

chronic high blood pressure, 213–214

chronic kidney disease (CKD), 31–32, 73–76
  defining, 74
  diagnosing, 74–75
  end-stage renal disease, 76–85
    dialysis, 77–82
    kidney transplant, 82–85
  nutrition plan for, 109
  staging and treating, 75–76

chronic obstructive pulmonary disease (COPD), 131

circle of Willis, 89

cirrhosis, 137

classifications, of blood pressure, 18

clinical studies, 185–189
  ACCORD trial, 188–189
  ADVANCE trial, 189
  SPRINT study findings, 186–187
  STEP trial, 187–188

clonidine, 171

clopidogrel, 93

coarctation of the aorta, 46

cognitive ability, 194–195

cold intolerance, 31

complete blood count (CBC), 22

complex carbohydrates, 127

compression socks, 202

computed tomography (CT) angiogram, 34, 96

computed tomography (CT) scan, 38, 96

congestive heart failure, 62–65
  determining underlying cause of, 63–64
  increasing risk of ARAS, 33
  signs and symptoms, 62–63
  treatment options, 65

congestive hepatopathy, 63

continuous ambulatory peritoneal dialysis, 78

continuous cycler-assisted peritoneal dialysis, 78

continuous positive airway pressure (CPAP) machine, 48

COPD (chronic obstructive pulmonary disease), 131

coronary angiography, 59

coronary artery bypass grafting (CABG), 61

coronary artery disease, 56–61
  angina and heart attack, 57–58
  diagnosing, 58–60
  minoxidil and, 177
  treatment options, 60–61
    angioplasty, 61
    bypass surgery, 61
    medication and lifestyle modifications, 60

cortisol, 42
  Cushing's syndrome, 43–45
  defined, 36

coumadin, 93

CPAP (continuous positive airway pressure) machine, 48

C-reactive protein (CRP), 58, 114

cross-country skiing, 148
CT (computed tomography) angiogram, 34, 96
CT (computed tomography) scan, 38, 96
Cushing's syndrome, 43–45
    diagnosing, 44–45
    treating, 45

D

D vitamin, 73
daily caloric needs, 116–118
dairy products, 111, 119, 126
dance, aerobic, 148
DASH diet, 108–114
    adjusting, 118–119
    adopting, 225
    foods and servings, 110–113
    leading up to, 108–109
    older people following, 199
    proving value of, 109–110
    reducing salt intake with, 113–114
DASH Diet For Dummies (Samaan, Rust, and Kleckner), 27
DASH-Sodium study, 110
DBP. *See* diastolic blood pressure
deep meditative breathing, 27, 151, 228
dehydration, 202
depression, 131, 171
detection, 13–22
    with accurate reading, 15–17
    classifications of blood pressure, 18
    having physical exam, 21–22
    looking at gauge used to measure, 14
    looking lab tests, 22
    lowering blood pressure too much, 19–20
    reviewing medical history, 21
    white-coat effect, 15
dexamethasone test, 45
diabetes, 19–20
    ACCORD trial, 188–189
    ADVANCE trial, 189
    beta blockers and, 172
    heart disease, 66–67
    reducing risk of, 128
    stroke, 92
Diabetes For Dummies (Rubin), 67, 92
diabetic neuropathy, 19–20

diabetic retinopathy, 104
dialysate, 78
dialysis
    hemodialysis, 80–82
    peritoneal dialysis, 77–80
dialyzer, 80
diastolic blood pressure (DBP), 9
    in children, 206
    classifications, of blood pressure, 18
    DASH diet reducing, 108
    in older people, 195
    overview, 17
diet, 107–120
    consulting with nutritionist, 120
    DASH diet, 108–114
    hemodialysis and, 82
    losing weight with nutrition, 115–119
        adjusting DASH nutrition plan, 118–119
        calculating ideal weight, 115–119
        determining daily caloric needs, 116–118
    Mediterranean diet, 114
    older people improving, 197–199
        assessing nutritional status, 198–199
        following DASH nutrition plan, 199
    plant-based diet plan, 115
discomfort, chest, 57
diuretics, 26, 65, 155–162
    aldosterone-antagonist diuretics, 161–162
    coming to market, 122
    loop diuretics, 158–160
    medication combinations, 163
    potassium-sparing diuretics, 160–161
    thiazide and thiazide-like diuretics, 155–158
dizziness, 19, 25, 31, 175
Doppler ultrasound tests, 97
dosages
    principles of, 177–178
    reducing, 30
doxazosin, 39, 175
dreams, disturbing, 171
dry mouth, 171

E

early delivery, 216
ECG (electrocardiogram), 58

echocardiogram, 59, 64, 90

e-cigarettes, 130

eclampsia, 216

ectopic Cushing's syndrome, 44

edema, 63, 75

ejection fraction (EF), 64

electrocardiogram (ECG), 58

electrolytes, 72

elevated blood pressure, 18, 205

embolectomy, 97

embolic stroke, 89

enalapril, 166

encephalopathy, 91

endarterectomy, 97

endocrinologists, 39

end-stage renal disease, 76–85

  dialysis, 77–82

    hemodialysis, 80–82

    peritoneal dialysis, 77–80

  kidney transplant, 82–85

energy drinks, 139

epinephrine, 130

  defined, 36

  pheochromocytoma, 37–39

  sympathetic nervous system using, 170

eplerenone, 162

eprosartan, 167

equipment, exercise, 147

erectile dysfunction, 156

erythropoietin, 73

essential high blood pressure, 9, 43

estrogen, 213, 219

ethacrynic acid, 159–160

ethnicity, 25–26

exercise, 65, 67, 141–152

  benefits of, 142

  for children, 208, 209

  complementary therapies, 149–152

    biofeedback, 151–152

    meditation, 150–151

    yoga, 150

  for gaining strength, 149

  for losing weight, 148

  myths about avoiding, 235

  predisposition for stroke and, 92

  preparing to begin program for, 142–147

    getting checkup, 143

    personalizing program, 144–147

    using right equipment, 147

  pushing blood back to heart, 202

  starting program, 227–228

eye exam, 22

eyes, 101–104

  anatomy of, 102

  hypertensive retinopathy, 103–104

F

facial weakness, 94

falls in blood pressure, 201–202, 212

family history, 25, 30

F.A.S.T. thinking, 94

fasting blood glucose, 115

fatigue, 172

fats, 55, 111, 119, 126

FDA (Food and Drug Administration), 124

felodipine, 169

fibromuscular dysplasia (FMD), 33

filtering, kidneys, 71–72

first-degree relatives, 25

fish, 111, 119

fistula, 80

fluid intake, 65

flushing spells, 30

FMD (fibromuscular dysplasia), 33

foam cells, 56

focal weakness, 87–88

Food and Drug Administration (FDA), 124

food labels, 124, 198, 226

fosinopril, 166

fructose, 127

fruits, 111, 119, 126

Fuhrman, Joel, 115

furosemide, 159

G

gauge, blood pressure, 14

genetics, 25, 206–207

genitourinary tract (GU tract), 70

gestational hypertension, 214

glucose, 53, 66–67

glycemic index, 128

golf, 148

grades, hypertensive retinopathy, 103

grains, 111, 119, 126

GU tract (genitourinary tract), 70

gum, nicotine, 135

H

Hatha yoga, 150

HDL (high density lipoprotein), 115

Headspace app, 151, 208

heart, 8

  overview, 52–53

  systole, 19

heart attack, 20

  myths about stopping medications after, 235

  overview, 57–58

  SPRINT study findings, 186

heart disease, 51–67

  blocking blood flow to heart muscle, 53–54

  caffeine and, 139

  cardiovascular system, 52–53

  congestive heart failure, 62–65

    determining underlying cause of, 63–64

    signs and symptoms, 62–63

    treatment options, 65

  coronary artery disease, 56–61

    angina and heart attack, 57–58

    diagnosing, 58–60

    treatment options, 60–61

  formation of plaque, 55–56

  risk factors, 65–67

    controlling diabetes, 66–67

    quitting smoking, 66, 131

    reducing high cholesterol, 66

    stepping up physical activity, 67

  SPRINT study findings, 186

heart exam, 22

heart failure, 20, 35, 186

heart medications, 20

heart muscle, 54

  blocking blood flow to, 53–54

  hypertrophy, 53

  inability to relax, 64

heart rhythm, 20, 90, 93

heartbeats, 63

heartburn, 139

heat intolerance, 31

HELLP syndrome (hemolytic anemia, elevated liver enzymes, and low platelets), 215

hematuria, 75

hemodialysis, 80–82

hemoglobin A1c, 67

high blood pressure, 7–11

  cardiovascular system, 8

  consequences of, 10

  detecting, 13–22

    with accurate reading, 15–17

    classifications of blood pressure, 18

    having physical exam, 21–22

    looking at gauge used to measure, 14

    looking lab tests, 22

    lowering blood pressure too much, 19–20

    reviewing medical history, 21

    white-coat effect, 15

  evaluating in children, women, and older people, 11

  global perspective of, 24

  lowering with different treatments, 10–11

  measuring blood pressure, 8–9

  myths about, 231–238

    aging and inevitability of high blood pressure, 231–232

    avoiding exercise, 235

    life restrictions, 233

    nervousness and anxiety, 237

    older people not needing treatment, 237

    stopping treatment after heart attack or stroke, 235

    stopping treatment if feeling good, 236

    taking medications forever, 234

    treatment for high systolic blood pressure, 234

    treatment is worse than disease, 232–233

    uncontrollable high blood pressure, 236–237

    women with high blood pressure, 238

  prevalence in United States, 1, 7

  risk factors, 9–10, 23–27

    changing lifestyle, 26–27

    ethnicity, 25–26

    genetics, 25

    medications, 26

high density lipoprotein (HDL), 115

high-fructose corn syrup, 127
high-salt foods, 125
Hispanics, 26
home hemodialysis, 80
home monitoring, 16–17
hormone replacement therapy (HRT), 219
hormones
  causing hypertension, 36–45
    detecting tumor that produces aldosterone, 39–43
    finding epinephrine-producing tumor, 37–39
    recognizing Cushing's syndrome, 43–45
  kidneys making, 72–73
  during pregnancy, 213
  women using, 218–219
    hormone replacement therapy, 219
    oral contraceptives, 218
HRT (hormone replacement therapy), 219
hydralazine, 176
hydrochlorothiazide, 157
hyperaldosteronism, 10, 39–43
  diagnosing, 40–42
  treating, 43
hyperinsulinemia, 115, 127
hyperlipidemia, 87
hypertension. *See* high blood pressure
hypertensive encephalopathy, 91
hypertensive retinopathy, 103–104
hyperthyroidism, 47
hypertrophy, 53, 63–64
hyponatremia, 200
hypothyroidism, 47

I

icons, in this book, 2
ideal weight, 115–119
idiopathic high blood pressure, 40
illegal drugs, 92, 207, 209
immunosuppressants, 84
impaired fasting glucose (prediabetes), 66
in-center hemodialysis, 80
incidentalomas, 42
indapamide, 157
infertility, 139
inhalers, nicotine, 135

inpatient rehabilitation unit, 99
insulin resistance, 21
intensity levels, exercise, 144–145
internal eye exam, 22
Intersalt Study, 122
intima, artery wall, 55
intravenous contrast, 34
irbesartan, 168
ischemia, 89
ischemic core, 97
ischemic penumbra, 97
isolated diastolic high blood pressure, 195
isolated systolic high blood pressure, 195

J

Journal of Clinical Hypertension, 123
Journal of Hypertension, 130

K

kidney disease, 25
kidney stones, 161
kidneys, 8, 69–85
  chronic kidney disease, 31–32, 73–76
    defining, 74
    diagnosing, 74–75
    staging and treating, 75–76
  end-stage renal disease, 76–85
    dialysis, 77–82
    kidney transplant, 82–85
  role of, 70–73
    filtering, 71–72
    making hormones, 72–73
kilocalorie, 148

L

lab tests, 22
  for Cushing's syndrome, 45
  screening for thyroid disease, 47
labetalol, 174
LDL (low-density lipoprotein), 55, 58
left ventricle hypertrophy, 53, 63–64
leg exercises, 202

legumes, 111

licorice, 42

lifestyle

  changing to prevent high blood pressure, 26–27

  children changing, 208–209

  coronary artery disease, 60

  exercise, 65, 67, 141–152

    benefits of, 142

    children with high blood pressure and strenuous, 209

    complementary therapies, 149–152

    for gaining strength, 149

    for losing weight, 148

    myths about avoiding, 235

    predisposition for stroke and, 92

    preparing to begin program for, 142–147

    starting program, 227–228

  modifications, 11

  older people modifying, 200

light in sodium label, 124

lightheadedness, 19, 25

lipid profile, 22, 66

lisinopril, 165

lithium, 159

long-acting nitrates, 60

loop diuretics, 158–160, 200

losartan, 168

low sodium label, 124

low-density lipoprotein (LDL), 55, 58

lowering blood pressure, 10–11, 223–230

  accurate blood pressure readings, 223–224

  adopting DASH diet, 225

  avoiding medications that raise blood pressure, 229–230

  cutting out caffeine, 225–226

  giving up tobacco and alcohol, 227

  knowing if you have resistant high blood pressure, 224–225

  older people avoiding dangerous falls, 201–202

  practicing mind-body techniques, 228–229

  reducing salt intake, 226–227

  starting exercise program, 227–228

  taking medications, 229

  too much, 19–20

low-salt diet, 126

lozenges, nicotine, 135

lumen, 56

lung cancer, 131

lung exam, 22

lupus-like syndrome, 176

M

macrophages, 55

magnesium, 109

magnesium sulfate, 216

magnetic resonance imaging (MRI) scan, 38, 96

Mayo Clinic Biofeedback Overview, 152

measuring blood pressure, 8–9

  accurate reading of measurement, 15–17, 223–224

  ambulatory readings, 17

  in children, 204–206

    interpreting results, 205–206

    on tiny arms, 204–205

meat, 111, 119, 126

medical history, 21

medications, 11, 153–184, 229

  allowing body to adapt to, 19–20

  brand names, 182–184

  children taking, 210

  choosing, 177–179

    adhering to prescription, 179

    personalizing choice, 178

    principles of medication dosing, 177–178

    selecting another medication when necessary, 178–179

  classes of, 154–177

    acting on nervous system, 170–175

    diuretics, 155–162

    first-line agents, 162–170

    vasodilators, 175–177

  congestive heart failure, 65

  coronary artery disease, 60

  diagnosing resistant high blood pressure by amount of, 29

  hormone replacement therapy, 219

  myths about

    stopping after heart attack or stroke, 235

    stopping if feeling good, 236

taking medications forever, 234

treatment is worse than disease, 232–233

treatment only needed for high systolic blood pressure, 234

older people taking

for lowering blood pressure, 200–201

for pain relief, 197

oral contraceptives, 218

raising blood pressure, 229–230

reducing dosage, 30

as risk factor, 26

side effects, 179–182

stroke, reducing risk of, 93

meditation, 27, 150–151, 228

Meditation For Dummies (Bodian), 151

Mediterranean diet, 114

men

global perspective of high blood pressure in, 24

heart attack in, 56

prevalence among different ethnicities, 25–26

MEN (multiple endocrine neoplasia), 39

mental-status examination, 194

mercury blood pressure gauge, 14

metabolic syndrome, 21, 115, 128

metanephrines, 38

methyldopa, 170–171

metolazone, 157–158

metoprolol, 173

microalbumin test, 22

migraines, 174

mind-body techniques, 228–229

Mini Mental State Examination (MMSE), 194

mini-stroke, 93, 94

minoxidil, 176–177

miscarriages, 139

moexipril, 166

monosodium glutamate (MSG), 124

Montreal Cognitive Assessment (MoCA), 195

Mountain Bike Review, 147

mouth cancer, 131

MRI (magnetic resonance imaging) scan, 38, 96

multiple endocrine neoplasia (MEN), 39

murmur, 46

myocardial infarction. *See* heart attack

myocardial perfusion scan (MPS), 58–59

N

nadolol, 173

narrowed renal arteries, 32–35

diagnosing renal artery stenosis (RAS), 33–34

treating blocked renal arteries, 34–35

nasal spray, nicotine, 135

National Center for Complementaty and Integrative Health, 149

National Heart, Lung, and Blood Institute, 205

neck examination, 22

nephrologists, 32, 75

nephrons, 72

nervous system, 170–175

nervousness, 237

neurologic conditions, 20

neurological exam, 22

neurotransmitters, 170

New England Journal of Medicine, 108, 225

nicotine, 130, 132, 227

Nicotine Anonymous, 136

nicotine replacement therapy, 135

nifedipine, 169

nitrates, long-acting, 60

nitroglycerin, 57, 60

no salt added label, 124

norepinephrine, 37, 170

normal blood pressure, 18

normetanephrines, 38

NSAIDS (nonsteroidal anti-inflammatory drugs), 26, 197, 230

nutrients, 8

Nutritarian diet, 115

nutrition

adjusting DASH nutrition plan, 118–119

calculating ideal weight, 116

determining daily caloric needs, 116–118

older people improving, 197–199

assessing nutritional status, 198–199

following DASH nutrition plan, 199

reducing salt intake, 199

nutritionists, consulting with, 120

nuts, 111, 119, 126

O

obesity, 92, 203
oils, 119
older people, 193–202
  assessing blood pressure in
    considering resistant high blood pressure, 196–197
    examining medications, 197
    recognizing baseline high blood pressure, 195
  avoiding dangerous falls in blood pressure, 201–202
  evaluating cognitive ability, 194–195
  evaluating in, 11
  improving nutrition to lower blood pressure, 197–199
    assessing nutritional status, 198–199
    following DASH nutrition plan, 199
    reducing salt intake, 199
  modifying lifestyle, 200
  myths about
    inevitability of high blood pressure, 231–232
    not needing treatment, 237
  taking prescription medications, 200–201
olmesartan, 168
1 alpha hydroxylase D, 73
online resources
  bike reviews, 147
  biofeedback equipment, 152
  body mass index calculations, 116
  cheat sheet for this book, 3
  DASH diet plans and recipes, 113
  devices evaluated for accuracy, 17
  Headspace app, 208
  help to quit smoking, 136
  National Center for Complementaty and Integrative Health, 149
  National Heart, Lung, and Blood Institute guidelines, 205
  Scientific Registry of Transplant Recipients, 85
  Silver Sneakers, 202
  social determinants of health, 24
  yoga, 150
ophthalmologists, 103
ophthalmoscope, 101
opiate pain medications, 20
optic disc, 102
oral contraceptives, 26, 218, 230
orthopnea, 62
orthostatic blood pressures, 186, 201

orthostatic hypotension, 20, 194
oscillometric blood pressure gauge, 187
  buying, 17
  overview, 14
osteoporosis, 139
outpatient rehabilitation unit, 99
overweight children, 203
oxygen, 8, 52, 130

P

palpitations, 31, 93
papilledema, 103–104
Parkinson's disease, 20
paroxysmal nocturnal dyspnea, 62
passive smoking (secondhand smoke), 131–132
patches, nicotine, 135
pedometers, 146
perceived exertion scale, 144–145
percentiles, 205
percutaneous coronary artery angioplasty (PTCA), 61
perindopril, 166
peripheral neuropathy, 137
peripheral vascular disease, 22
peritoneal dialysis, 77–80
peritoneum, 77
peritonitis, 80
pharmacy blood pressure readings, 14
phenoxybenzamine, 39
pheochromocytoma, 37–39
physical exam, 21–22
plant-based diet plan, 115
plaque, formation of, 53, 55–56
plasma renin activity, 207
postpartum preeclampsia, 216
potassium chloride, 123
potassium level, 31, 34, 109, 123, 156
potassium-sparing diuretics, 160–161
poultry, 111
prazosin, 175
prediabetes (impaired fasting glucose), 66
preeclampsia, 214–217
pregnancy, 156, 212–218
  ACE inhibitors during, 164
  after delivery high blood pressure, 217–218
  angiotensin II receptor blockers, 167

beta blockers during, 172

causes of high blood pressure during, 213–217

nifedipine, 169

premenstrual pain, 139

prepared foods, 226

pressure sensors, 202

primary hyperaldosteronism. *See* hyperaldosteronism

progesterone, 213

prolactin, 213

propranolol, 173–174

prostate medications, 20

protein, in urine, 217

proteinuria, 74–75

pseudo high blood pressure, 196

PTCA (percutaneous coronary artery angioplasty), 61

pulse

in arteries, 22

rapid, 31

Q

quinapril, 166

Quitting Smoking & Vaping For Dummies (Elliot and Smith), 133

R

rales, 63

ramipril, 167

RAS (renal artery stenosis), 33–34

reduced sodium label, 124

relapsing, 133–134

relaxation, 151

relaxin, 213

relaxing, heart muscle, 64

renal arteries, 71

renal artery Doppler ultrasound, 34

renal artery stenosis (RAS), 33–34

renal cortex, 71

renal pyramids, 71

renal vascular hypertension, 32

renin, 32, 34, 72–73, 213. *See also* hyperaldosteronism

resistant high blood pressure, 29–48

caffeine amounts and, 138

coarctation of the aorta, 46

considering chronic kidney disease, 31–32

hormones causing hypertension, 36–45

detecting tumor that produces aldosterone, 39–43

finding epinephrine-producing tumor, 37–39

recognizing Cushing's syndrome, 43–45

hyperthyroidism and hypothyroidism, 47

narrowed renal arteries, 32–35

diagnosing renal artery stenosis, 33–34

treating blocked renal arteries, 34–35

in older people, 196–197

reducing blood pressure and knowledge of, 224–225

signs and symptoms of, 30–31

sleep apnea, 47–48

retina, 102

risk factors, 9–10, 23–27

changing lifestyle, 26–27

children

hereditary influences, 206–207

weight, 207

ethnicity, 25–26

genetics, 25

heart disease, 65–67

controlling diabetes, 66–67

quitting smoking, 66

reducing high cholesterol, 66

stepping up physical activity, 67

medications, 26

stroke, 92–93

Road Bike Review, 147

rubber bulb, 14

running, 148

S

salivary cortisol test, 45

salt sensitivity. *See also* sodium intake

overview, 123–124

in women, 212

SBP. *See* systolic blood pressure

Scientific Registry of Transplant Recipients, 85

secondary high blood pressure. *See* resistant high blood pressure

secondhand smoke (passive smoking), 131–132

sedentary lifestyle, 142

seeds, 111, 119, 126

serum chemistry profile, 22

servings, DASH diet, 110–113

shared decision making, 193–194
side effects
  ACE inhibitors, 164
  beta blockers, 172
  recognizing common, 179–182
  spironolactone, 162
  thiazide diuretics, 156
Silver Sneakers, 202
simple carbohydrates, 127
sinus rhythm, 90
skilled nursing facility, 99
sleep, 139
sleep apnea, 21, 47–48
sleepiness, 171
slurred speech, 94
smokeless tobacco, 132
smoking, 27
  children, 209
  heart disease, 66
  taking oral contraceptives and, 218
smoking-cessation aids, 135–136
smooth muscle, 176
SNS (sympathetic nervous system), 170
snuff, 132
social determinants of health, 24
sodas, 139
sodium free label, 124
sodium intake, 27, 65, 121–126
  connection between high blood pressure and, 122
  kidneys regulating, 72
  lowering
    avoiding high-salt foods, 125
    children, 209
    with DASH diet, 113–114
    going on low-salt diet, 126
    reading food labels, 124
    suggestions for, 226–227
  role of potassium, 123
  salt sensitivity
    overview, 123–124
    in women, 212
sphygmomanometer, 14
spironolactone, 43, 162
SPRINT (Systolic Blood Pressure Intervention Trial), 18, 186–187
stable angina, 57

stage 1 high blood pressure, 18
stage 2 high blood pressure, 18
staging, chronic kidney disease, 75–76
standing up, 19–20
stents, 35, 61, 97
STEP (Strategy of Blood Pressure Intervention in the Elderly Hypertensive Patients), 187–188
steroids, 230
strength training, 144, 149
stress management, 208
stress test, 58
stretch marks, 31
stroke, 87–99
  causes of
    atherosclerosis, 88–89
    brain hemorrhage, 90–91
    cerebral embolus, 89–90
  myths about stopping medications after, 235
  preventing, 91–93
    with medications, 93
    risk factors, 92–93
  recovering from, 98–99
  SPRINT study findings, 186
  thinking F.A.S.T., 94
  treatments, 97–98
  utilizing brain imaging, 95–97
Stroke For Dummies (Marler), 88
subarachnoid space, 90
sucralfate, 159
sugar, 65
  connection between high blood pressure and, 127
  reducing risk of metabolic syndrome and diabetes, 128
sulfa medications, 156
supermarket blood pressure readings, 14
sweets, 111, 119, 126
swimming, 148
sympathetic nervous system (SNS), 170
systole, 19
Systolic Blood Pressure Intervention Trial (SPRINT), 18, 186–187
systolic blood pressure (SBP), 9
  in children, 206
  classifications, of blood pressure, 18
  DASH diet reducing, 108
  myths about treatment with high, 234
  in older people, 195

overview, 17
SPRINT study, 186–187
STEP trial, 187–188
systolic heart failure, 64

T

tachycardia, 37–38
taste sensation, 199
telmisartan, 168
tennis, 148
terazosin, 175
therapies, 149–152, 228–229
  biofeedback, 151–152
  meditation, 150–151
  for stroke rehabilitation, 99
  yoga, 150
thiazide and thiazide-like diuretics, 155–158, 165, 196, 200
thinking F.A.S.T., 94
throat cancer, 131
thrombectomy, 97
thrombotic stroke, 89
thyroid disease, 47
Thyroid For Dummies (Rubin), 47
TIA (transient ischemic attack), 93, 94
ticagrelor, 93
tissue plasminogen activator (tPA), 97
tobacco, 130–136
  accelerating atherosclerosis, 93
  avoiding all forms of, 132
  consequences of using, 131, 227
  examining extent of problem, 130–131
  quitting successfully, 133–136
  reducing exposure to secondhand smoke, 131–132
torsemide, 160
tPA (tissue plasminogen activator), 97
transcendental meditation, 151
transdermal estrogen, 219
transient ischemic attack (TIA), 93, 94
transplant, kidney, 82–85
treatments, 10–11
  chronic kidney disease, 75–76
  congestive heart failure, 65
  coronary artery disease, 60–61
  hyperaldosteronism, 43

pheochromocytoma, 39
  stroke, 97–98
triamterene, 161
triglycerides, 115
troponin levels (cardiac enzymes), 58
tumors
  epinephrine-producing, 37–39
  producing aldosterone, 39–43
type 2 diabetes, 188

U

ulcers, 139
unsalted label, 124
unstable angina, 57
ureter, 70
urethra, 70
uric acid levels, 156, 168
urine
  decreased, 63
  indicating kidney problem, 75
  protein in, 217
  test, 38, 45

V

valsartan, 168
valsartan-neprilysin, 65
vaping, 130, 207, 209
varenicline, 136
vascular disease, 33
vasodilators, 175–177
vegetables, 111, 119, 126
vegetarians, 108–109
veins, 8
vena cava, 52
ventricles, 19, 52
very low sodium label, 124
Voltaren, 197

W

waist circumference, 21, 115, 118
walking, 145–146, 148, 227
waste products, 8
water aerobics, 148

water retention, 197

weight loss, 65, 115–119

  adjusting DASH nutrition plan, 118–119

  calculating ideal weight, 115–119

  children, 207, 208–209

  determining daily caloric needs, 116–118

  exercise for, 148

  unintentional, 198

white-coat effect, 15, 206, 224

withdrawal, 229

without added salt label, 124

women, 211–217

  connecting high blood pressure and salt sensitivity in, 212

  evaluating high blood pressure in, 11

  global perspective of high blood pressure in, 24

  heart attack in, 56

  myths about having high blood pressure, 238

  pregnancy and high blood pressure, 212–218

    causes of during, 213–217

    dealing with after delivery, 217–218

  prevalence among different ethnicities, 25–26

  using hormone treatments, 218–219

    hormone replacement therapy, 219

    oral contraceptives, 218

Y

yoga, 27, 150, 228

Yoga Basics, 150

Yoga Journal, 150

Yoga with Adriene, 150

About the Author

Richard W. Snyder, DO, has been treating and studying high blood pressure and kidney disease for the past two decades. He is an author of *Medical Dosage Calculations For Dummies* and is dedicated to improving the lives of those with high blood pressure and kidney disease. He has also been involved in graduate medical education for more than 15 years and has taught physicians, medical residents, medical students, and advanced practitioners. He continues to treat patients who have high blood pressure and kidney disease and is committed to using a holistic approach to the treatment of high blood pressure, with an emphasis on nutrition, lifestyle modifications, and medications when needed.

Dedication

This book is dedicated to my mother, Nancy, a nurse who has dedicated her life to improving the physical and spiritual health of others. She is a constant source of inspiration. I hope she knows the significant impact she has had on my life.

Author's Acknowledgments

I would very much like to acknowledge several individuals. First, I would like to thank my wonderful editor, Elizabeth Kuball. I very much thank her for her guidance and help in creating this important book. She is a master of the written word. I would also like to acknowledge my friend and colleague, Dr. Mahesh Krishnamurthy, who served as technical editor for this book. He was a constant source of encouragement regarding the book, and that's truly appreciated. I also would like to acknowledge Dr. Alan Rubin, who wrote the first two editions. He is truly a great writer and physician, and I appreciate the opportunity to be a part of this journey. I also want to thank Tracy Boggier and Vicki Adang for their help and encouragement regarding this book. To all of them, I owe major thanks.

Publisher's Acknowledgments

Senior Acquisitions Editor: Tracy Boggier

Editor: Elizabeth Kuball

Technical Editor: Mahesh Krishnamurthy, MD

Production Editor: Pradesh Kumar

Illustrator: Kathryn Born, MA

Cover Image: © fcafotodigital/Getty Images

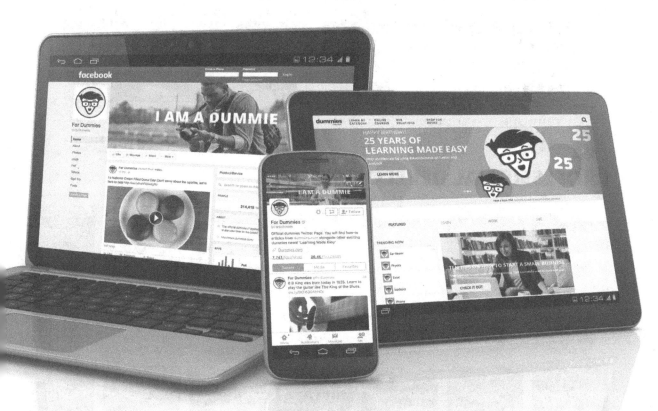

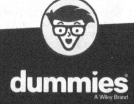

PERSONAL ENRICHMENT

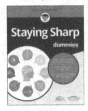

Staying Sharp
9781119187790
USA $26.00
CAN $31.99
UK £19.99

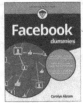

Facebook
9781119179030
USA $21.99
CAN $25.99
UK £16.99

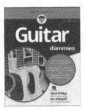

Guitar
9781119293354
USA $24.99
CAN $29.99
UK £17.99

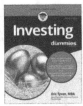

Investing
9781119293347
USA $22.99
CAN $27.99
UK £16.99

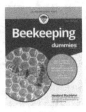

Beekeeping
9781119310068
USA $22.99
CAN $27.99
UK £16.99

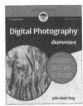

Digital Photography
9781119235606
USA $24.99
CAN $29.99
UK £17.99

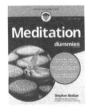

Meditation
9781119251163
USA $24.99
CAN $29.99
UK £17.99

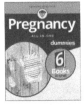

Pregnancy
9781119235491
USA $26.99
CAN $31.99
UK £19.99

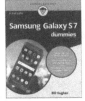

Samsung Galaxy S7
9781119279952
USA $24.99
CAN $29.99
UK £17.99

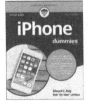

iPhone
9781119283133
USA $24.99
CAN $29.99
UK £17.99

Crocheting
9781119287117
USA $24.99
CAN $29.99
UK £16.99

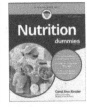

Nutrition
9781119130246
USA $22.99
CAN $27.99
UK £16.99

PROFESSIONAL DEVELOPMENT

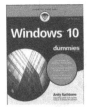

Windows 10
9781119311041
USA $24.99
CAN $29.99
UK £17.99

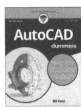

AutoCAD
9781119255796
USA $39.99
CAN $47.99
UK £27.99

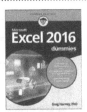

Excel 2016
9781119293439
USA $26.99
CAN $31.99
UK £19.99

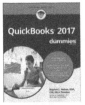

QuickBooks 2017
9781119281467
USA $26.99
CAN $31.99
UK £19.99

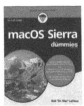

macOS Sierra
9781119280651
USA $29.99
CAN $35.99
UK £21.99

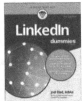

LinkedIn
9781119251132
USA $24.99
CAN $29.99
UK £17.99

Windows 10
9781119310563
USA $34.00
CAN $41.99
UK £24.99

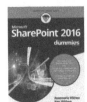

SharePoint 2016
9781119181705
USA $29.99
CAN $35.99
UK £21.99

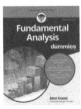

Fundamental Analysis
9781119263593
USA $26.99
CAN $31.99
UK £19.99

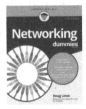

Networking
9781119257769
USA $29.99
CAN $35.99
UK £21.99

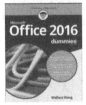

Office 2016
9781119293477
USA $26.99
CAN $31.99
UK £19.99

Office 365
9781119265313
USA $24.99
CAN $29.99
UK £17.99

Salesforce.com
9781119239314
USA $29.99
CAN $35.99
UK £21.99

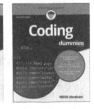

Coding
9781119293323
USA $29.99
CAN $35.99
UK £21.99